ULTRASONIC IMAGING and ANIMAL REPRODUCTION: FUNDAMENTALS

BOOK 1

by

O. J. GINTHER, VMD, PhD

Professor of Veterinary Science

University of Wisconsin
1655 Linden Drive
Madison, WI 53706

1995

Library of Congress Catalog Card No. 94-072805

ISBN 0-9640072-3-1

Published and distributed by:

Equiservices Publishing
4343 Garfoot Road
Cross Plains, WI 53528 USA
Phone or Fax: 608-798-4910

to

my graduate students—past and present—
who have or will become
independent and productive biologists

Preface to the Original Book

Ginther, O. J. 1986. *Ultrasonic Imaging and Reproductive Events in the Mare.* Equiservices Publishing, Cross Plains, Wisconsin, USA.

No one was prepared—nor could they have been. The proliferation of ultrasound scanners in equine theriogenology in the early 1980s was unexpected. The availability of a real-time noninvasive technology for visualizing internal structure and content of the reproductive organs generated enthusiasm and high expectations. Purchase costs exceeded \$20,000. Today, costs exceed \$10,000, which is still a considerable sum. Unless a durable, high-quality scanner is purchased and reasonable use is made of its capabilities, a fair return on investment may not be attained. This book should help practitioners and researchers make an appropriate decision regarding purchase. Those who already have a scanner will be able to expand and sharpen their techniques. Even if one does not have access to a scanner, much information can be gained from this text; ultrasonic morphology is thoroughly integrated with gross anatomy, histology, physiology, endocrinology, and pathology. Moreover, recent research findings obtained with the help of ultrasonic imaging are reviewed. These findings add the dimension of dynamics to our understanding and appreciation of the beauty of equine reproductive function. It will be seen that dynamics—active motions and forces—are essential in the functioning of the reproductive tract. The book is intended for research scientists and graduate students as well as clinicians and veterinary students. Except for introductions, the book progresses from one expanded legend to another without the use of intervening text. It is, in effect, an elaborate slide show. This format eliminates the nuisance and discontinuity associated with searching for tables and figures.

Preface

This series of books is an outgrowth of *Ultrasonic Imaging and Reproductive Events in the Mare* published in 1986. The series will eventually involve reproductive ultrasonography in many animal species. The fundamentals that apply to all species are covered in Book 1, including principles, equipment, image interpretation, and techniques of ultrasonic imaging of the reproductive tracts of animals. In addition, a chapter on research considerations is included. Book 2 is devoted to equine reproductive ultrasonic imaging, and Book 3 will involve the nonequine large-animal species (cattle, goats, llamas, pigs, sheep, large zoo animals). The series approach is being used to allow purchase flexibility, since many animal scientists and veterinarians are dedicated to certain species.

In keeping with the style of the original book, the text, in effect, progresses from figure legend to figure legend and thereby eliminates the nuisance of searching for figures and tables. In almost all instances, the reader can study the textual information and the related figure without turning a page. A second feature involves the manner in which the book is tied together as follows: 1) notations in the text regarding other pages in the text of closely related information, 2) notations in the Summary on the pages of the detailed information, and 3) notations in the Bibliography to direct the reader to pages where each reference is cited. These unique features were possible because the author and word/figure processor worked side-by-side as the book evolved. The goal was to produce a series of books conducive to pleasurable reading, researching, and browsing.

This book series is supplemented by an independently available 50-minute video tape. The videotape provides a real-time perspective on ultrasonic imaging of the dynamic reproductive tract and also features animated demonstrations involving principles and interpretation.

Acknowledgments

Some of the experiments reviewed in this series of texts were done during thesis research, including the preparation of many of the sonograms. The following graduate students made extensive use of ultrasound scanners: Gregg Adams, Don Bergfelt, Chris Bessent, Karin Bodensteiner, Laurence Bonafos, Elaine Carnevale, David Cross, Sandy Curran, Eduardo Gastal, Pat Griffin, Karen Hayes, John Kastelic, Gayle Leith, Roger Pierson, Stan Scraba, and David Townson. Thanks are also extended to Krzysztof Kot, Cathy Miller, and Debra Williams for ultrasonic scanning, Lisa Kulick for illustrative work, Tom Roberts for preparation of photographs, Ellen Dodge Severson for editorial help, and Jane Ginther of Equiservices Publishing for word processing and typesetting. Thanks are extended to John Parks, ultrasound coordinator at the University of Wisconsin Hospital, for preparing the sonograms from the Acuson scanner. Some photographs of equipment were made from equipment at the School of Veterinary Medicine and the School of Medicine at the University of Wisconsin and from scanners borrowed from Classic Medical Supply. Photographs of their equipment were provided by Cooke Veterinary Products and Products Groups International.

CONTENTS

Part One

PRINCIPLES

Part Four

SUMMARY

Part Five

APPENDIX

Part One

PRINCIPLES

Chapter 1

INTRODUCTION

Gray-scale, real-time ultrasonography is the most profound technological advance in the field of animal research and clinical reproduction since the introduction of transrectal palpation and radioimmunoassay of circulating hormones (author's opinion). Veterinary students in some schools are still being taught that ultrasound is a secondary technology for large-animal reproduction work—an adjunct to transrectal palpation. This is not realistic. The information-gathering capabilities of ultrasonic imaging far exceed those of palpation, except for consistency and sensitivity, which require the tactile sense. Ultrasonography provides non-invasive information on the internal anatomy of the reproductive organs and their payload, the conceptus. Dramatic events can be seen while they are occurring, and apparently without interference. A high point in the author's career occurred when a Day-14 equine embryo approached a cyst in the middle of the uterine body, encroached upon it with appropriate distortion of the conceptus, squeezed over the cyst, continued moving in the same direction until it reached the cervix, and then reversed direction. This event happened during a six-minute span and was observed and photographed as it occurred. It is not surprising to hear veterinarians say that ultrasound scanners are the spice in their practice. They're fun.

But ultrasonography is a complex, expensive technology in which the operator, scanner, and tissues must interact to produce a useful, pleasing image. The first major thrust of this book (Part 1) is to provide a thorough working knowledge of the principles of ultrasound, so that the operator-scanner interaction is optimal and the financial investment receives maximal return. Once suitable images of an area of interest are obtained, the next step is interpretation—relating the ultrasonic information to tissue structure, and thereby reaching a conclusion. The representation of tissue structure by both factual and artifactual echoes is considered in depth. The second thrust (Part 2) involves the selection and operation of the instruments and techniques of examination. Integration of the technology into research programs is considered in Part 3. A summary is presented as Part 4 and provides page information for locating details. The appendix (Part 5) includes information on sources of equipment and supplies, as well as a comprehensive bibliography and subject index.

An Overview

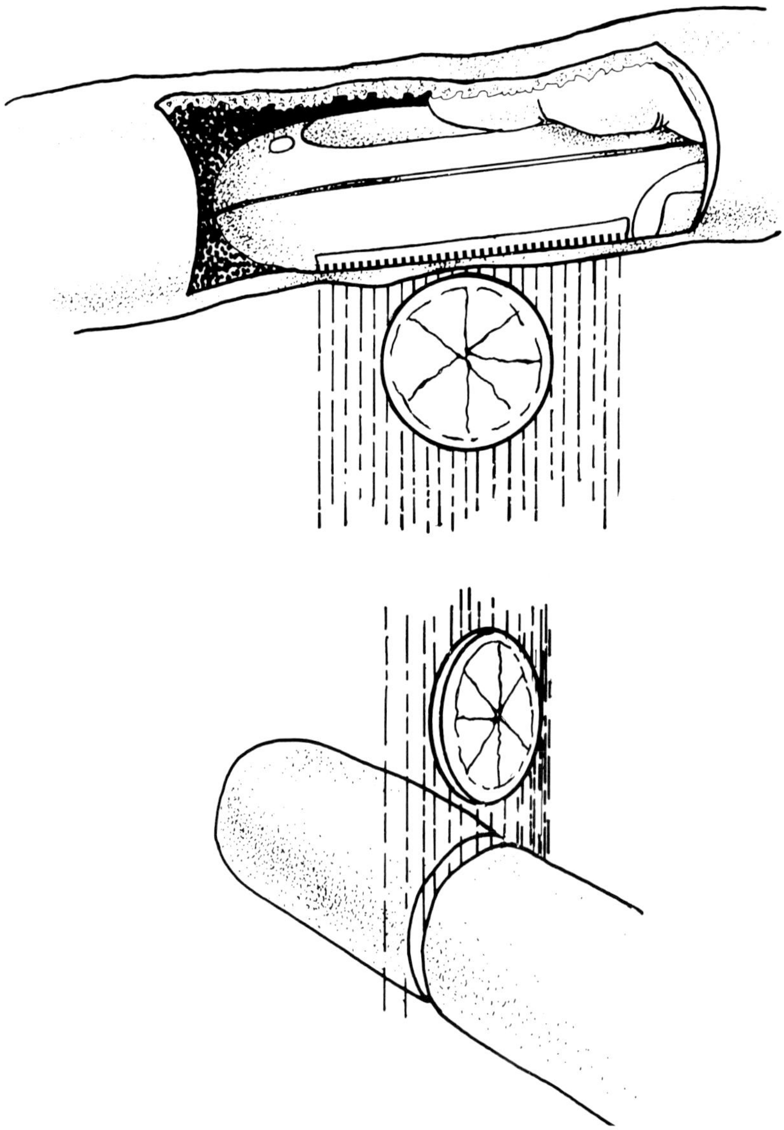

Sampling a cross-sectional "slice" of uterine horn. In the larger species (cattle, horses), the remote unit of an ultrasound system (transducer) can be hand held in the rectum directly over the organs of interest, as shown. In smaller species (sheep, goats, dogs), a rigid extension can be fastened to the intrarectal transducer for external manipulation, or the transabdominal route can be used. Diagnostic ultrasound uses high-frequency sound waves to produce images of soft tissues and internal organs. Electric current is applied to crystals in the transducer, producing vibrations characteristic of the crystals and resulting in sound waves. The operator directs the sound waves through the tissues by moving or varying the angle of the transducer. Close proximity of rectal or abdominal wall to the organs allows the use of high-frequency scanners that produce images with much detail. The sound beams that pass through the tissues are quite thin (e.g., 2 mm) in the focal area, and a thin "slice" of tissue is sampled, as shown. The two-dimensional image seen on the screen is analogous to a histologic section.

Tissues have different abilities to either propagate or reflect sound waves. The proportion of the sound wave that is reflected is received by the transducer, converted to electric impulses, and displayed as an echo on the ultrasound screen. The characteristics of various tissue interfaces determine what proportion of the sound wave will be reflected. The reflected portion is represented on the ultrasound image by shades of gray, extending from black to white. Liquids (follicular fluid, yolk-sac fluid) do not reflect sound waves and are said to be nonechogenic or anechoic; therefore, the image of a liquid-containing structure appears black on the screen. Dense tissues (cervix, fetal bone) reflect much of the sound beam and appear white (echogenic) on the screen. Other tissues are seen in various shades of gray depending upon their echogenicity. Certain tissue formations may cause the sound waves to bend or bounce back and forth or to become weakened or entirely blocked. Therefore, artifacts appear on the screen and will challenge the interpreting abilities of the ultrasonographer.

Modern ultrasound instruments for examining the reproductive tract of animals are B-mode, real-time scanners. B-mode refers to brightness modality, in which the ultrasonic imaging is a two-dimensional display of dots. The brightness of the dots is proportional to the amplitude of the echoes. Real-time imaging refers to the moving display in which the echoes are recorded continuously, and events such as fetal-leg movements and heartbeat can be observed as they occur. Most scanners have videotaping capabilities so that the moving images can be preserved. They may be played back through the ultrasound scanner or a television set. The moving image also can be "frozen" to facilitate study, measurements, or photographic reproduction.

Studying "living," detailed, sequential, sectional views of the organs demands a working knowledge of anatomy more extensive than that required for palpation. Specialists in animal reproduction have entered an era in which they must be knowledgeable not only in gross and histologic anatomy and pathology, but also in ultrasonic anatomy and pathology. They must be able to relate the image on the viewing screen to normal and abnormal form and function.

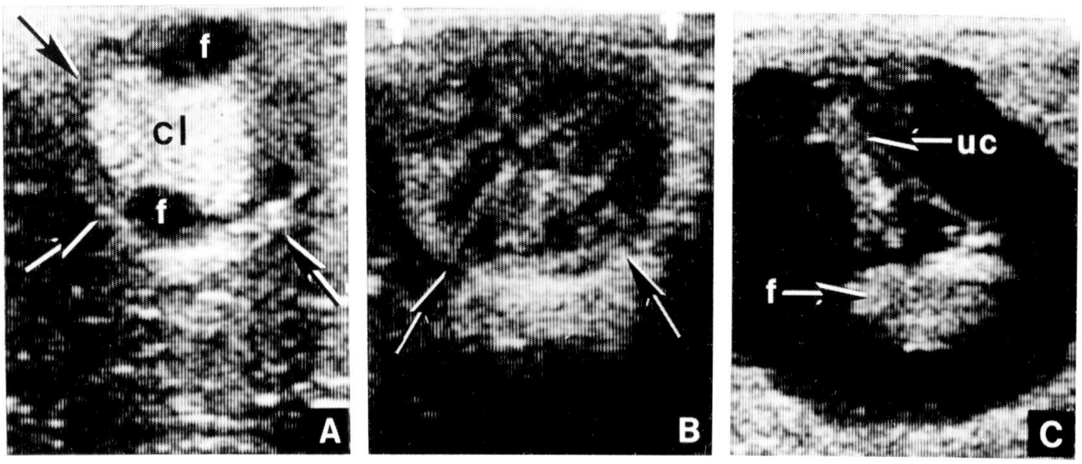

Examples of ultrasound images. The images were taken with a 5 MHz linear-array transducer from the reproductive tract of mares and are intended as an introduction to gray-scale imaging.

(A) Ultrasonic slice of an ovary. The ovary, delineated by arrows, has a corpus luteum (cl) and two 8 to 10 mm follicles (f). The corpus luteum is beginning to regress and is very dense and therefore highly echogenic.

(B) Image of a cross-section of a uterine horn taken during estrus. The lower edge of the horn is delineated by arrows. The edematous endometrial folds are prominent. The center of each fold is more reflective and therefore relatively echogenic (light gray or white), whereas the outer portions are relatively anechoic (dark gray or black).

(C) Day-45 conceptus. Allantochorionic fluid is black (anechoic), whereas the tissues are shades of gray (f=fetus; uc=umbilical cord).

Note the various shades of gray, extending from black to white. The shade depends on the proportion of the sound wave that is reflected back to the transducer—the more reflected, the lighter the shade of gray. The reflecting surfaces are called tissue interfaces. An interface results wherever tissues of different density are in contact. Uniform areas, such as the fluid of a structure (follicles, allantochorion) do not reflect sound waves and are said to be nonechogenic or anechoic. Fluid is therefore dark or black on the images. The various tissues are white or shades of gray, depending on their echogenicity (ability to reflect sound waves). The interfaces of denser structures are more reflective and numerous, resulting in a whiter image.

Clinical Uses

When introduced to the veterinary reproduction field, transrectal ultrasound scanners were used primarily in mares for early pregnancy diagnosis, detection of twins, and photographic documentation of pregnancy. Ultrasonic scanners have now assumed a broader, more fundamental role in equine reproductive management, clinical diagnosis and monitoring, and the technology has been extended to most of the common animal species. Detailed information on the many uses of ultrasound in evaluating and monitoring reproductive structures and events in animals will be given in later books of this series. The following list highlights some specific clinical uses:

1. Determining the seasonal status of the ovaries.
2. Determining whether a female has reached puberty.
3. Monitoring follicles for diagnoses or assessing treatments.
4. Differentiating single and double ovulatory follicles and ovulations.
5. Establishing time or failure of ovulation.
6. Monitoring the corpus luteum.
7. Estimating the stage of the estrous cycle.
8. Differentiating luteal persistence from anovulatory conditions.
9. Estimating the extent of endometrial estrogen exposure.
10. Evaluating the time and suitability for breeding.
11. Detecting semen in the uterus.
12. Collecting follicular oocytes by transvaginal aspiration.
13. Evaluating an animal's potential to serve as an embryo-transfer recipient.
14. Detecting and studying the early embryo.
15. Detecting twin embryos and, in mares, manually eliminating one.
16. Diagnosing twins (twin membrane) during the later fetal stage.
17. Determining fetal sex.
18. Assessing fetal viability and prepartum position.
19. Evaluating postpartum uterine involution.
20. Diagnosing precise time of embryonic death (absence of heartbeat).
21. Diagnosing ovarian pathologic conditions such as luteal and follicular cysts, peri-ovarian cysts, ovarian tumors, and hemorrhagic follicles.
22. Diagnosing pathology of tubular organs such as hydrosalpinx, pyometra, uterine cysts, and collections of intraluminal uterine fluid and fetal debris.

Evolution of Animal Reproductive Sonography

Ultrasonic real-time imaging in animal reproduction has a short history. The following list of full-length original reports is intended to illustrate the expanding acceptance and utility of B-mode, real-time ultrasonic imaging. A few reports are preceded by an asterisk to indicate potential milestones in the evolving utilization of real-time imaging:

1980 * First report of transrectal imaging of the reproductive tract in large animals (mares; *117*).

Ultrasonography promoted as a diagnostic tool in animals with a notation on detecting the canine prostate *(28, 29)*.

Early 1980s Rapid increase in the use of transrectal ultrasound by equine theriogenologists *(35, 114, 139, 150)*.

1982 Transrectal ultrasonic pregnancy diagnosis in cattle *(34)*.

1983 Detailed descriptions of ultrasonic anatomy of the embryo and utero-embryo interactions in horses *(51, 52)*.

First in a series of in-depth reviews on ultrasonic evaluation of the reproductive tract of mares *(55, 78, 81)*.

Transabdominal sonographic evaluation of the prostate *(32)* and pregnancy in dogs *(20)*.

Transabdominal ultrasonic pregnancy diagnosis in pigs *(91)*.

Short course on the use of ultrasound to evaluate the equine reproductive tract (Colorado State University).

Introduction of 5 MHz intrarectal linear-array transducers for reproductive studies in animals *(78)*.

1984 * Use of ultrasonic imaging for studying the changing follicular populations in horses *(80)* and cattle *(123)*.

Detailed descriptions of ultrasonic anatomy of ovaries *(80)* and nongravid and postpartum uterus *(79)* in horses.

Report that the equine embryo is detectable ultrasonically by Day 9 or 10 and almost always by Day 11 *(55)*.

Use of ultrasonic detection of small intrauterine fluid collections to diagnose metritis in horses *(2, 58, 71, 79)*.

First reports on imaging of the ovary, including luteal cavities and superovulatory response *(123)*, and embryonic development *(122)* in cattle *(142)*.

Transabdominal ultrasonic detection of ovulation in dogs *(90)*.

Transabdominal ultrasonic pregnancy diagnoses in sheep *(173)*.

1985 Transrectal ultrasonic pregnancy diagnosis in sows *(30)*.

First use of ultrasonically detected simulated biological structures (equine embryo) for reproduction research in any species *(56)*.

Detailed ultrasonic studies of preovulatory follicle *(125)*, corpus luteum *(124)*, and natural *(66)* and induced *(57)* embryonic death in horses.

1986 * First text and reference book on ultrasonic imaging in animal biology (reproductive tract of mares; *58*).

Ultrasonic studies of the embryo and fetus *(40, 41)*, uterine pathology *(49)*, spontaneous embryonic loss *(33, 40)*, luteal cavities *(98)*, and placentomes *(41)* in cattle.

Transrectal ultrasonic pregnancy diagnosis in sheep *(24)*.

Ultrasonic fetal gender diagnosis using the scrotum and mammary glands in large animals (cattle; *112*).

Transabdominal ultrasonic evaluation of reproductive disease in dogs *(133)*.

Transcutaneous ultrasonic assessment of testes in boars *(31)*.

Transabdominal ultrasonic pregnancy diagnoses in cats *(43)*.

1987 * First report on ultrasonic assessment of uterine contractility in any species (horses and donkeys; *37*).

Transcutaneous ultrasonic assessment of testes in bulls *(119)*.

Ultrasonic morphology of the nongravid *(128)* and postpartum *(116)* uterus in cattle.

* First continuous ultrasonic monitoring of the ovulatory process in any species (horses; *164*).

Transrectal ultrasonic assessment of accessory sex glands in stallions *(102)*.

1988 * First reports on sonographic monitoring of the growth and regression profiles of individual follicles throughout the estrous cycle in any species (cattle; *129, 147, 152*).

Reviews on imaging of the ovaries and uterus *(129)* and the conceptus *(95)* in cattle.

* Transvaginal imaging for viewing the internal genitalia and for ultrasonically guided aspiration of oocytes in animals (cattle; *131*).

Transrectal ultrasonic assessment of accessory sex glands in bulls *(170)*.

1989 Ultrasonic morphology of genital tract in female llamas *(1)*.

* First reports of computerized pixel analyses as an aid in reproduction research in any species (horses; *165, 167*).

Use of ultrasound to teach and evaluate AI technicians in cattle *(13)*.

Compilation of reviews on ultrasonic imaging in animal reproduction *(159)*.

Intrauterine presentation and accessibility of fetus in cattle as determined by transrectal ultrasonography *(93)*.

Ultrasonic study of the growth and regression of individual follicles in horses *(151)*.

* First use of the location of the genital tubercle for early diagnosis of fetal gender in any species (cattle and horses; *38, 39*)

1990 Ultrasonic study of the growth and regression of individual follicles in llamas *(5)*.

Transrectal ultrasonic pregnancy diagnosis in red deer *(17)*.

Ultrasonic assessment of testes and sperm output in stallions *(103)*.

Sonographic study of pregnancy in dolphins *(175)*.

1991 Ultrasonic study of fetal dynamics and uterine-diameter dynamics in horses *(84)*.

* Detailed descriptions on the feasibility of transrectal imaging in endangered species, including early detection (27 days after breeding) of the embryo in the rhinoceros *(4)*.

Ultrasonic morphology of the corpus luteum in llamas *(6)*.

First use of artificial echogenic markers in reproduction research in any species (horses; *84*).

* First ultrasonic study of accessory sex glands during ejaculation in any species (horses; *171*).

1992 First detailed report of research techniques and adaptability of transrectal imaging to research in reproductive biology *(85)*.

Temporal relationships between ultrasonically detected follicular waves and FSH surges in cattle *(3)* and horses *(14, 67)*.

Ultrasonic diagnosis of seminal vesiculitis in stallions *(105)*.

Ultrasonically guided, transvaginal aspiration of follicular oocytes in horses *(23, 36)*.

1993 Ultrasonic assessment of follicles in sheep *(148)*.

Detection of ovulation by ultrasound in pigs *(153)*.

Use of the ultrasound technique for study of fetal presentation changes *(73)*, allantoic fluid shifts, and uterine horn closures *(62)* in horses.

First report of ultrasonically guided cannulation for sampling ovarian venous blood in animals (cattle; *113*).

First ultrasonic assessment of follicular waves in prepubertal animals in any species (cattle; *46*).

1994 Sonographic detection of a twin membrane for diagnosis of twin fetuses in mares *(74)*.

Review of ultrasonic studies on equine utero-fetal kinetics *(64)*.

Ultrasound studies of follicular waves in goats *(77)* and pigs *(145)*.

Study of the buffalo conceptus by transrectal ultrasound *(118)*.

1995 Ultrasonic assessment of uterine contractility in cattle *(19)*.

Temporally associating ultrasonically detected follicular waves with FSH surges in sheep *(76)*

In 1980, one hundred years after the discovery of the piezoelectric effect, Palmer and Driancourt *(117)* described the use of a hand-held 3 MHz intrarectal transducer and real-time gray-scale scanner for monitoring reproductive events in mares, and Cartee *(28, 29)* described ultrasonography as a new diagnostic technique in veterinary medicine. Their pioneering work opened the way for the increasing use of real-time ultrasonography in animal reproduction. Several reports given at the 1982 International Symposium on Equine Reproduction generated excitement over the potential of the technique. In 1982-84, research and clinical reports began to appear that described in detail the transrectal ultrasonic anatomy and pathology of the reproductive tracts of mares and cows and the transabdominal ultrasonic appearance of pregnancy and the prostate in dogs. The interest in the technology soon led to the development of the first short course in reproductive ultrasonography (Colorado State University, E. L. Squires and associates). Sufficient interest and information was available by 1986 to justify a text and reference book on the narrow subject of transrectal diagnostic ultrasonography of the reproductive tract of mares. In retrospect, this was the first book on sonography in veterinary medicine, illustrating the major role played by equine theriogenologists and reproductive biologists in the adaptation of diagnostic ultrasound to the veterinary and animal research fields. Subsequent developments of historical note include the adaptation of the technology for diagnosing fetal sex, collecting follicular oocytes, and studying the dynamics of accessory sex glands, growth profiles of individual follicles, and uterine contractility.

General 100-year History

A brief outline of the early history of the development of diagnostic ultrasound *(9, 176)* is given below:

1880 Discovery of the piezoelectric effect.

1940s Refinement of SONAR (SOund NAvigation and Ranging).

Ultrasonic detection of flaws in metals.

SONAR equipment used to demonstrate echoes deep within body tissues.

1950s Echo-encephalography and echocardiography in humans.

Water-path scanner.

1960s Contact scanner.

Two-level (black and white) images.

1970s Electronic scan converter and gray-scale imaging.

Real-time ultrasound in humans.

A-mode and Doppler ultrasound for pregnancy diagnoses in animals.

1980 Introduction of real-time imaging to the animal field.

Without the discovery of the piezoelectric properties of certain crystals, diagnostic ultrasonography would not have evolved. It is this property that permits the conversion of electric current to ultrasound waves and the subsequent conversion of the mechanical energy of echoes into electric current. The research activities necessitated by World War II led to the refinement of SONAR, in which ultrasound waves were used to detect submarines. This principle was then slowly adapted to the detection of tissue reflectors.

The earliest systems for abdominal and pelvic imaging used a water-path scanner, a medical extension of the SONAR technique in which the patient was seated in a tank of water. The submerged transducer moved in a circle around the patient. The contact scanner represented an important advance, because the transducer could be applied directly to the subject without passage of the sound waves and echoes through a water bath. A layer of gel between the skin surface and the transducer served to eliminate air, which would have blocked the passage of the ultrasound waves.

Older scanners in the 1960s used a system in which the wide range of echo amplitudes was compressed into two levels, so that various parts of the image were either black or white. This approach was limited because it defined only major differences in tissue densities. The development of gray-scale imaging in the early 1970s was a major advance. Many amplitudes of echoes were represented by levels of the gray scale. The signals were stored in a scan converter and then displayed on a television monitor. The original analog converters have been replaced by digital scan converters, which store the echo information (location, amplitude) in a memory similar to that used in personal computers. The digital scan converters were more stable and more resistant to electronic noise.

Another major breakthrough was real-time or dynamic imaging, which became available in the late 1970s. This approach allowed the operator to observe movements (e.g., heartbeat, moving fetal limbs) as they occurred. Among other things, the viability of an embryo could be established immediately. As far as animal reproduction is concerned, a one-hundred-year history of ultrasound began in 1880 with the discovery of piezoelectric crystals and extended to 1980, when the technology of B-mode, real-time ultrasonic imaging was introduced to the animal field.

A Revolutionary Research Tool

Animal and veterinary scientists are only beginning to realize the tremendous potential of ultrasonography as a research tool. Totally unsuspected discoveries already have been made, and the technology is being used for conventional scientific testing of hypotheses. Many research areas now being investigated by the use of ultrasonography were once largely inaccessible. The research ramifications of ultrasonic imaging for investigating reproductive events will be discussed in Chapter 9. In large-animal reproduction research, use of ultrasonic imaging has resulted in the following discoveries:

1983 Mobility *(52)* and fixation *(51)* of early equine embryos.

1984 Dynamic interactions between twin equine embryos *(53)*.

Occurrence of natural reduction in unilateral, but not bilateral, equine twin embryos *(54)*.

1985 Ultrasonic morphology of endometrial folds as an instant biological indicator of estrogen levels during the estrous cycle and the reproductive seasons in horses *(87)*.

Physical nature of early embryonic loss in horses, including documentation of expulsion through cervix *(57, 66)*.

Failure of many equine corpora lutea to develop as corpora hemorrhagica *(124)*.

1986 Sequential changes in follicular populations in cattle *(126)*.

1987 Greater spiraling of the bovine uterine horns during diestrus than during estrus, contrasting to perceptions based on palpation *(128)*.

Sequential changes in follicular populations in horses *(127)*.

Duration and patterns or types of follicular evacuation during ovulation in horses *(164)*.

Contrasts in uterine contractility during the embryo mobility phase versus the estrous cycle stages in horses *(37)*.

1988 The phenomenon of periodic development of dominant and subordinate follicles (cattle; *129, 147, 152*).

1989 Compartmentalization of the gravid bovine uterus *(94)*.

Reduction of equine twin embryos by one-way deprivation *(60)*.

Morphologic resurgence of the primary corpus luteum during pregnancy in horses *(15)*.

Retention and eventual expulsion through the cervix, rather than resorption, of debris following embryonic loss in cattle *(96)*.

Discharge during ovulation of most follicular fluid into the abdomen, rather than oviduct, in horses *(166)*.

Straightening and curling of uterine horns during estrus and diestrus, respectively, in llamas *(1)*.

1990 Follicular waves in llamas *(5)*.

1991 Changing diameter of uterine horns during the estrous cycle and early pregnancy in horses *(84)*.

Periodic transient constrictions of the gravid uterus and resulting allantoic-fluid shifts in horses *(84)*.

1992 Relationships between emergence of follicular waves and FSH surges in cattle *(3)* and horses *(14, 67)*.

Minor as well as major follicular waves in horses *(63, 67)*.

1993 Delayed emergence and reduced number of follicles in the ovulatory follicular wave in old mares *(70)*.

Reclosure of uterine horns in mid-pregnancy and close encasement and retention of the fetal hind limbs by the umbilical-cord horn until parturition in horses *(62)*.

Local effect of equine embryo on uterine contractions and morphology *(86)*.

1994 Natural outcome of twins during the early fetal stage in horses *(74)*.

Follicular wave phenomenon in goats *(77)*.

Defective óocytes in old mares as determined with the aid of transvaginal ultrasonically guided instrumentation *(27)*.

Follicular waves in sheep and the temporal association with FSH surges *(76)*.

Other Modes

Although the diagnostic ultrasonography described in this text involves the B-mode for real-time two-dimensional imaging, other modes are available for study of soft tissue *(138)*.

The A-mode (amplitude mode) produces a one-dimensional display of echo amplitudes for various depths, depicted as a line graph; the axes are amplitude and depth. The A-mode is in widespread use for evaluating the fat and lean portions of meat animals and also has been used for pregnancy diagnosis (pg 139). In the late 1970s, A-mode machines were overpromoted for diagnosis of pregnancy in small animals, sheep, and horses. The unsuitability of these machines for this purpose, especially in horses, resulted in some resistance to the real-time, B-mode scanners when they were introduced to the veterinary market in the early 1980s; prospective buyers tended to recall their unfavorable experiences with the A-mode machines.

The M-mode (motion mode) form of imaging is an adaptation of the B-mode and is used for evaluating moving structures such as the heart. The change in reflector depth at various times is displayed as a simple line graph; the axes are depth and time.

Doppler ultrasound systems (pg 109) use the motion of blood toward, away, or at an angle to the transducer to construct dazzling multicolor images of flow patterns (e.g., red=toward transducer; blue=away from transducer; mixture of colors=turbulence). The Doppler effect for auditory sound is often illustrated by the changes in sound frequency as a train approaches and leaves an observer. Ultrasonic Doppler systems were used during the 1970s and early 1980s for pregnancy diagnoses, especially in dogs and sheep (pg 138).

Duplex scanners combine real-time imaging with pulsed Doppler or with the M-mode. With such instrumentation, a vessel can be located with a real-time linear or convex transducer (pg 109). The Doppler mode can then be activated to study the blood flow. For example, an internal vascular area can be delineated, and the device will then provide an accurate measure of blood velocity in the designated vessels.

Side Effects

Although detrimental biological effects of ultrasonic imaging have not been reported for animals *(58)*, the possibilities of adverse effects must be diligently and continuously evaluated. If adverse tissue effects are eventually demonstrated, the findings will likely be well-publicized. Meanwhile, those with interest in the status of recent studies in this highly technical and important area can consult recent reviews *(18, 25, 48, 99, 161)*.

Concerns about the technology's side effects are heightened upon consideration of the delicate internal details of cells together with the responses of tissue to ultrasound waves (vibration of tissue molecules, absorption of heat). Such concerns seem especially warranted when considering rapidly growing, dividing, or highly functional or active cells, such as those in the ovaries (oocytes, follicular cells, luteal cells) and, most notably, in an embryo or fetus. The interaction of ultrasound with cells or tissues includes thermal and cavitation mechanisms. However, thermal effects with diagnostic ultrasound are apparently inconsequential; it is believed that temperature elevations would not reach 1 degree Celsius. Cavitation, a non-thermal mechanism involving an interaction with tiny gas bubbles, is capable of disrupting cells and tissues. Cavitation has been demonstrated with in vitro ultrasound experiments, but there have been no reports of cavitation in connection with in vivo diagnostic ultrasound examination.

Exposure to ultrasound is measured in units of intensity and duration. The minimum intensity (pg 29) required to produce a measurable effect on tissues is 100 milliwatts/Cm2; the tissues must be exposed for hours. Profound harmful effects have been reported in laboratory animals and in in vitro studies at these intensities and duration. However, diagnostic ultrasound scanners emit only 1 to 10 milliwatts/Cm2; apparently no observable effects have been confirmed at these intensities, even when animals or tissue were exposed much longer than for diagnostic examinations.

The American Institute of Ultrasound in Medicine has stated the following *(25)*:

> No confirmed biological effects on patients or instrument operators caused by exposure at intensities typical of present diagnostic ultrasound instruments have ever been reported. Although the possibility exists that such biological effects may be identified in the future, current data indicate that the benefits to patients of the prudent use of diagnostic ultrasound outweigh the risks, if any, that may be present.

Other Information Sources

Recent reviews on real-time ultrasonic imaging of the reproductive tract of animals include the following:

Horses *59, 109, 110, 111, 130, 141, 155, 159*
Cattle..................................... *22, 95, 129, 130*
Sheep, goats, pigs.......... *100, 144, 157, 159*
Dogs, cats........................... *11, 158, 177*

A review of the research applications of ultrasonic imaging in large animal reproductive biology was published in 1992 *(85)*, followed by an update in 1994 *(65)*. Short courses in ultrasonography have become common (pg 196), a reflection of demand, and are routinely announced in professional journals such as the Journal of the American Veterinary Medical Association, Journal of Equine Veterinary Science, and Veterinary Record.

The American Institute of Ultrasound in Medicine (AIUM) holds annual meetings, including an animal section, and distributes instructional material (source information: pg 196). The AIUM has videotapes of reports given at its conventions and has videotapes of an educational series including the following courses: 1) gynecologic ultrasound, 2) color Doppler ultrasonography, and 3) animal ultrasound. Special courses with videotapes and slides are also available from the Radiological Society of North America (source information: pg 196). The Ultrasound Quarterly publishes review papers on sonography, including an occasional paper in the animal field (e.g., small animals, *177*; horses, *141*).

Readers who develop a special interest in the animal ultrasound technology should be aware of the Veterinary Ultrasound Society. Its official newsletter, "Ultratalk," is published periodically in the journal, Veterinary Radiology and Ultrasonography. The journal has included articles on ultrasonic imaging since 1981, and in 1992 the journal began to include "ultrasonography" in its title *(162)*. The expansion of the journal title reflects the growing popularity of this imaging technology.

A 50-minute videotape on the principles, interpretation, and power of ultrasonic imaging of the reproductive tract in animals *(72)* is available from the distributors of this book (source information: pg 196). The videotape can be considered supplementary to this book because of the real-time imaging, colored animations, and taped demonstrations of techniques in various animal species. Other instructional videotapes are available (source information: pg 196).

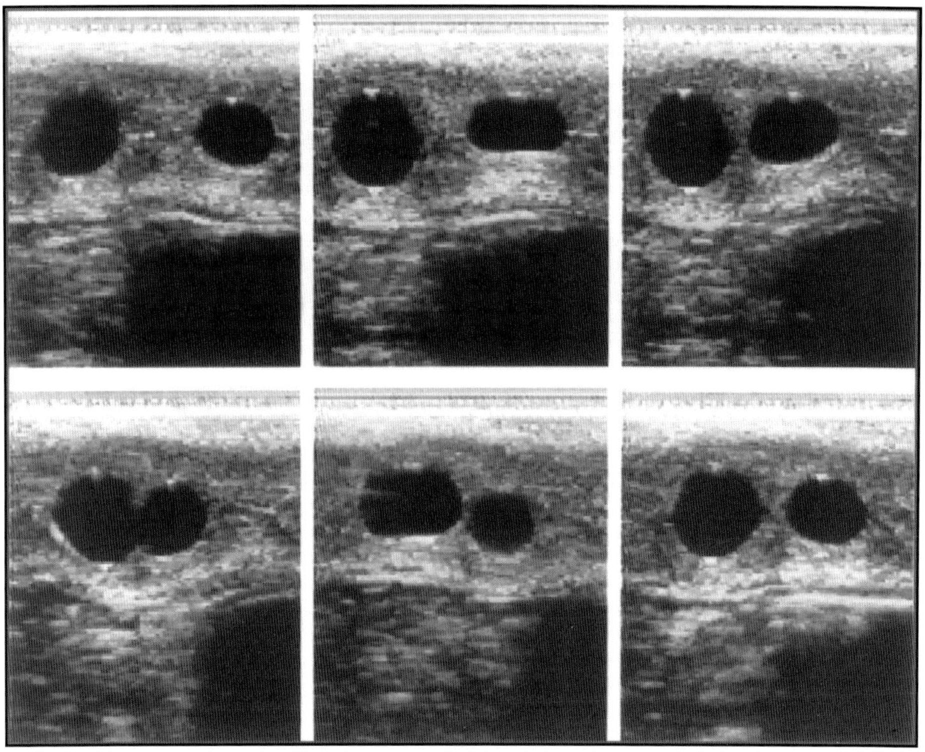

Playtime

Dynamics of Day-13 and Day-14 twin equine embryonic vesicles in response to uterine contractions. The series encompasses 17 seconds from first to last sonogram.

Chapter 2

WAVES AND ECHOES

Descriptions and discussions of the physical principles of diagnostic ultrasound are incorporated into Chapters 2 to 5. These discussions are simplified and represent the minimal exposure to ultrasound physics required for attaining optimal and pleasurable use of this technology. The information was gleaned from the highly technical and detailed presentations that were cited in the original book *(58)*. The cited texts were intended for ultrasonographers and physicians in human medicine, and cursory examination of the reports, including the complex mathematical formulas and symbols, should reveal the extent of simplification used here. The information in the original book has been updated and modified by perusal of recent text and reference books *(25, 47, 48, 83, 106)*. Additional resources included ultrasound physicists and specialists at the University of Wisconsin Medical School and electrical engineers, promotional literature, and specifications from animal ultrasound companies. The concepts were modified where indicated, and the diagrams were designed to relate directly to ultrasound scanners being used to examine the reproductive tract of animals.

In this chapter, background information is developed on the nature of ultrasound waves and echoes. This is done by comparing the origin, traveling, and echoing of audible sound in air with the origin, traveling, and echoing of ultrasound in tissues. The origin of audible sound from a drumhead, traveling of the resulting waves through air, echoing of the waves from a mountain side, reception of the echoes by the ear drum, and processing of the ear-drum vibrations by the internal auditory system are compared with the origin of ultrasound from transducer crystals, traveling of the resulting waves through tissue, echoing of the waves from tissue reflectors, reception of the echoes by the transducer crystals, and processing of the crystal vibrations by the ultrasound scanner.

Sound Waves

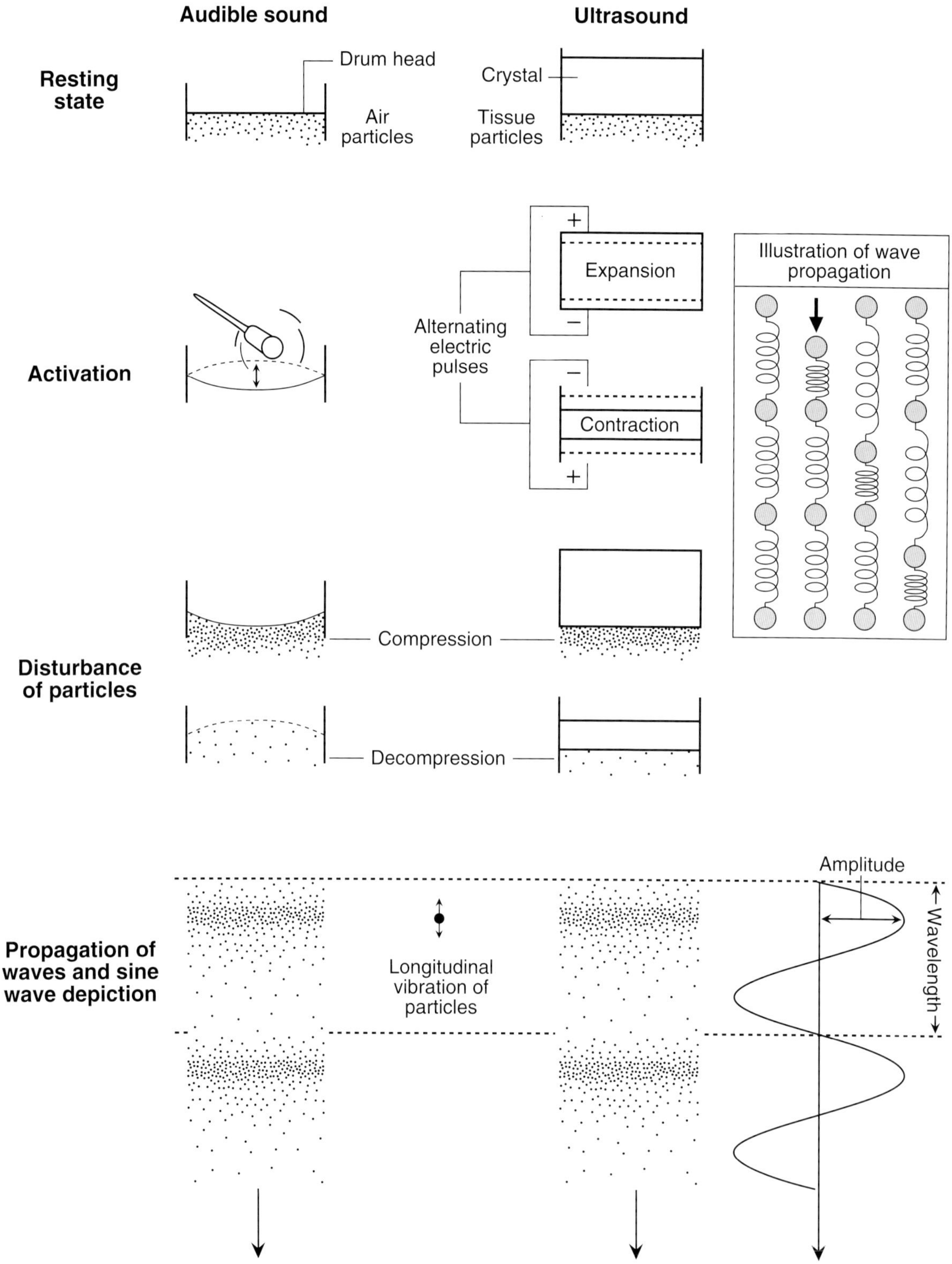
Audible sound
Ultrasound
Resting state
Drum head
Air particles
Crystal
Tissue particles
Activation
Alternating electric pulses
Expansion
Contraction
Illustration of wave propagation
Disturbance of particles
Compression
Decompression
Propagation of waves and sine wave depiction
Longitudinal vibration of particles
Amplitude
Wavelength

Comparison between audible sound waves and ultrasound waves (facing page). In this example, audible sound is produced by a diaphragm stretched over a hoop, as in a drumhead. During the resting state, the drumhead is still. The adjacent air particles or molecules are evenly dispersed and maintain an equilibrium due to mutually attracting and repelling forces. However, when the drumhead is activated by striking, it vibrates and disturbs the adjacent air particles. As the drumhead moves in one direction, it causes compression among the particles. When the drumhead moves in the opposite direction, it creates a void or decompression. In comparison, diagnostic ultrasound originates from crystals that have piezoelectric properties. Piezoelectric means literally "squeeze-electric." The crystals expand and contract when subjected to an electric current and, conversely, produce an electric current when compressed by returning echoes. A crystal is activated by an electric charge, which causes expansion or contraction of the crystal according to the alternating polarity of the electric signal. Crystal expansion causes compression among neighboring tissue particles, and contraction causes decompression similar to the response of air particles near the drumhead. In audible sound, the vibrating drumhead causes a disturbance of air particles in the form of alternating compression and decompression passing through the air away from the drumhead. It is the disturbance of the air particles that is propagated—not the particles themselves. The air particles vibrate and the oscillations are longitudinal in the direction of the sound wave. Similarly, ultrasound waves are mechanical pressure waves that are propagated through tissue by the alternating expansion and contraction of the piezoelectric crystal in response to the alternating polarity of the electric signal.

To visualize energy propagation, imagine that particles are separated by springs in equilibrium, just as neighboring particles in tissue are separated by equal repelling and attracting forces (see boxed illustration; *25*). An impact (arrow) on the first particle causes compression of the first spring. The compression is then transferred to the next spring and the first spring undergoes decompression. In association with the compression and decompression of springs, the particles move correspondingly (vibrate).

The bottom portion of the figure shows the association between the propagated waves of compression and decompression and the conventional method of diagrammatically depicting waves. Amplitude refers to the strength or power of the sound waves and is similar to volume or "loudness" in audible sound systems. Intensity refers to the rate of energy flow through a unit area in association with propagation of the sound waves and involves the rate of particle vibration. Intensity measurements are often used in discussions of possible biological effects of ultrasound (pg 24). Amplitude and intensity are directly related. A wavelength is the distance encompassed by an area of compression and the accompanying area of decompression and is depicted as a sine wave. Frequency refers to the number of vibrations or oscillations of the sound source (drumhead or ultrasound crystal) per second. It is therefore identical to the number of wavelengths or cycles that pass a given point in the medium per second, and to the number of vibrations made by the particles in the medium per second. Frequency is measured in hertz (Hz) units. One hertz is one cycle per second and a megahertz (MHz) is one million cycles per second. Ultrasound is defined as any sound with a frequency of more than 20,000 Hz. Diagnostic ultrasound uses frequencies of 1 to 10 MHz. Recently designed equipment for detailed study in ophthalmology, for example, uses frequencies of 10 to 25 MHz. Velocity is the time required for a wavelength to pass a given point. Velocity is determined by the characteristics of the medium (elasticity and density). In soft biological tissue, velocity averages approximately 1540 meters/second, excluding bone (4080 m/sec) and lung tissue (600 m/sec because of air). That is, ultrasound waves travel through tissue at approximately 1.5 millimeters in one millionth of a second. Although these complexities and characteristics should be kept in mind, sound waves will be depicted as simple arrows in some of the diagrams that follow.

The characteristics of sound waves resulting from a drumhead and those resulting from an ultrasound crystal were depicted in the above illustration on the same scale for didactic purposes. However, the two types of sound differ profoundly. For example, audible sound and ultrasound, respectively, differ as follows: 1) wavelength, 2 to 2000 cm versus <1 mm;; 2) frequency, 20 to 20,000 Hz versus 1 to 10 MHz; and 3) velocity, 330 m/sec versus 1540 m/sec. High-frequency ultrasound waves, unlike audible sound waves, tend to behave like a directed beam rather than spreading out during propagation. This important characteristic allows the ultrasonographer to precisely locate small reflectors deep within the tissue; two small reflectors can be differentiated only when the space between them is greater than the width of the beam or ultrasound pulses (pg 46). The heterogeneous nature of the medium for ultrasound (tissue), in contrast with the more homogeneous nature of the medium for audible sound (air), causes extensive interaction with the passage of ultrasound waves. As described in subsequent chapters, it is these interactions that are fundamental to diagnostic ultrasonography.

Reception of Echoes

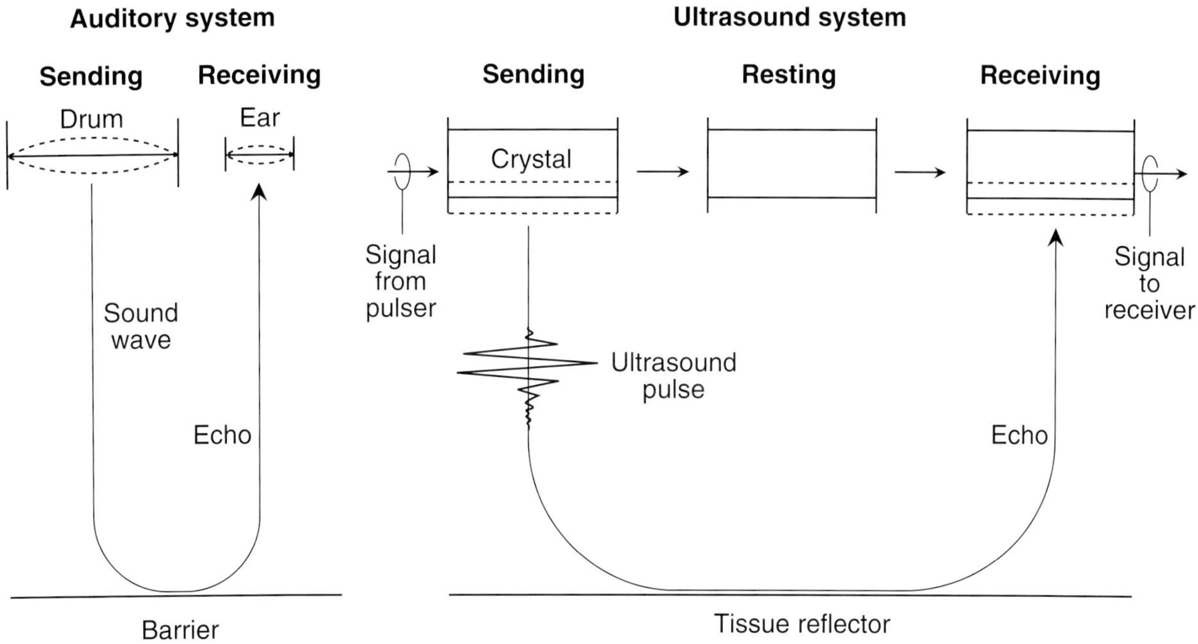

Comparison of the reception of echoes from audible sound and diagnostic ultrasound. The audible sound from the drumhead is propagated, getting weaker as it travels. If a barrier, such as a mountain, is reached before the sound becomes too weak, the sound is reflected or echoed in the same frequency and speed as in its production at the drumhead. The returning echo impinges on an ear drum, producing vibrations of the ear drum that are interpreted by the listener's internal auditory system. The distance between the drumhead and the barrier can be estimated on the basis of the known velocity of audible sound in air. Similarly, an ultrasound wave travels through the body tissue until it reaches a tissue reflector. Some of the sound is reflected and returns to the crystal. The force of the returning sound wave compresses and expands the crystal, which produces a voltage that is transmitted to a receiver. As noted above, the piezoelectric property of the crystal is such that it can both generate ultrasound waves when charged with an electric signal and generate an electric signal when struck by the returning ultrasound waves. The delay between propagation of the wave and reception of the echo is used to determine the distance from the crystal to the reflector.

Attenuation

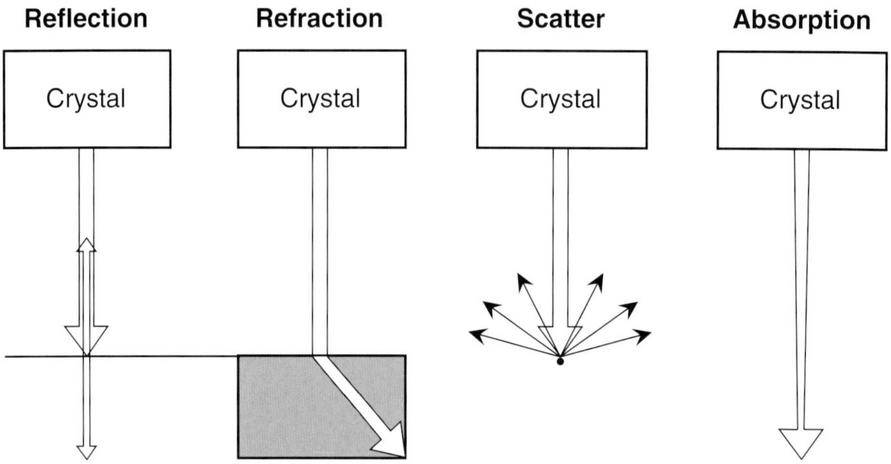

Causes of attenuation of ultrasound waves as they pass through tissue. Attenuation is defined as progressive weakening in intensity of the ultrasound waves as they travel through tissue, thereby limiting the depth of penetration. Body tissue is a complex medium, and ultrasonic waves in tissue therefore undergo complex modifications. The heterogeneous nature of tissues results in tissue interfaces wherever tissues of different density are in contact. Density imparts a quality known as acoustic impedance, which is a measure of the resistance to the propagation of sound waves. Acoustic impedance relates to the ultrasonic compressibility and stretchability of a tissue. Dense structures have particle density and low compressibility and are said to have high acoustic impedance. It takes only a small difference in density to result in an interface.

When ultrasound waves cross a perpendicular interface, a portion of them is returned to the transducer in the form of a reflection or echo. If the interface is not perpendicular, the pulses will be reflected at an angle (pg 66). The magnitude of the difference in acoustic impedance between the tissues on each side of the interface determines how much of the waves will be reflected. Usually only a small amount is reflected, and the remainder interacts with other interfaces deeper in the tissue. Often the most interesting echoes arise from interfaces that differ only slightly in acoustic impedance (1% or less). However, the difference in impedance is sometimes so great that most of the wave is reflected. For this reason, one cannot "see" through a soft tissue and air interface. The tissue-gas interface may result in reflection of more than 99% of the wave. This occurs commonly in ultrasonic examination of the reproductive tract due to air pockets in the intestines. It is noteworthy that the proportion reflected is not altered by increasing the amplitude of the waves. Air is also a troublesome barrier when trapped between the crystals and the tissue being examined. For this reason, a coupler or gel may be applied between the crystals and the skin in preparation for a transabdominal examination. In addition, it may be necessary to clip the hair to minimize air pockets. A gel is not needed when the surface of the tissue is wet and excludes air between the crystals and the tissue surface.

Refraction represents another interaction of ultrasound and tissue. Refraction refers to the bending of the sound waves as they cross tissues or fluids with different acoustic properties. Refraction occurs only when the tissue interface is not perpendicular to the ultrasound waves *(25)*. This is comparable to the bending of a light beam as it passes from air into water. Bending decreases the intensity of the returning echoes and therefore contributes to attenuation. This phenomenon is common in imaging of the reproductive tract because of the prevalence of curved surfaces of fluid-filled structures (e.g., follicles, embryonic vesicles, cysts). Even the slight difference in the speed of sound between soft tissue and fluid is enough to cause refraction. Refraction is of considerable importance to the ultrasonographer because refraction and reflection cause a common artifact in which a distinct shadow appears below the lateral edges of fluid-filled structures.

Scatter occurs when a sound wave encounters an interface that is irregular or smaller than the wavelength. Scatter is very important in imparting ultrasonic textures that are characteristic for a given tissue. It is the same process that highlights a beam of light traveling through dust-laden air *(134)*.

Absorption occurs when tissue captures the energy of the sound waves. Most of this energy is converted to heat and is the basis for ultrasound diathermy, a common use of therapeutic ultrasound. In diagnostic ultrasound, however, low energy levels are involved, and the biological effect of absorption is negligible (pg 24). Absorption is the only process that directly removes energy from the ultrasound waves; the other factors (reflection, refraction, scatter) redirect all or some of the wave front.

Production of Pulses

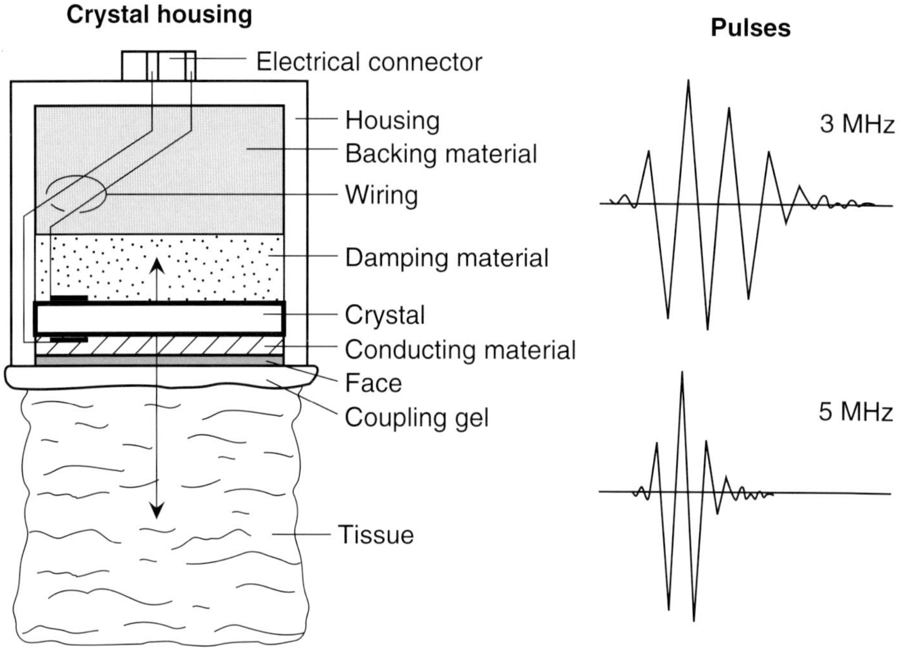

Housing of the crystal and method of damping the crystal vibrations for the production of short pulses. The active unit (piezoelectric crystal) is housed in an element assembly, as illustrated for a single-crystal unit. The face of the crystal is covered with conducting materials to favor the passage of the ultrasound waves into the tissue and also the pickup of the small voltages produced by the returning echoes. This conducting, or matching, layer has an impedance between those of the transducer crystal and the tissue. Therefore, it reduces reflection at the element-tissue interface and improves sound transmission through the interface. Wires run from the external electric connector to the crystal and conduct the relatively large voltages needed for crystal excitation, as well as the small voltages produced by the echoes. The housing of the assembly is connected to a grounding system. The plastic cover and facing shields the animal from the voltages needed to excite the crystal. The crystal is subjected to a short series of electric excitations, resulting in a short series of vibrations known collectively as a pulse. The resulting energy is generated in both directions, as shown by the arrows. The crystal is backed by a highly energy-absorbent damping material.

The damping process absorbs the energy above the crystal and quickly reduces the vibrations. As a result, a well-defined burst or pulse of waves is produced, that travels through the gel coupler and into the medium.

The short, pulsed nature of the generated waves allows an interval of quiescence to permit reception of potential echoes by the same crystal. For example, the pulse of waves might be 2 to 3 mm in length and contain four cycles. The frequency of ultrasound crystals is so great that 1,000 pulses, each consisting of 3 or 4 cycles, may be emitted per second despite the requirement that there be a pause between pulses for echo detection. The damping process produces nearly the same number of vibrations, regardless of frequency of the crystal. Therefore, as shown on the right, a higher-frequency crystal (e.g., 5 MHz) has the same number of waves per pulse, but the pulse is shorter than that of a lower-frequency crystal (e.g., 3 MHz). These relationships are the basis for one of the tenets of ultrasound—higher frequency results in better resolution. Because of the vital role of damping, the quality of an ultrasound image is influenced by the design of the damping process, as well as by crystal frequency.

The speed of the gathering of echo information should be appreciated. Transmission of a pulse and collection of the resultant echoes are completed in about 0.25 milliseconds. That is, 4000 pulses or lines of echo information can be collected in one second. If, for example, 100 lines of information are needed to complete an image, 40 images are generated per second *(106)*.

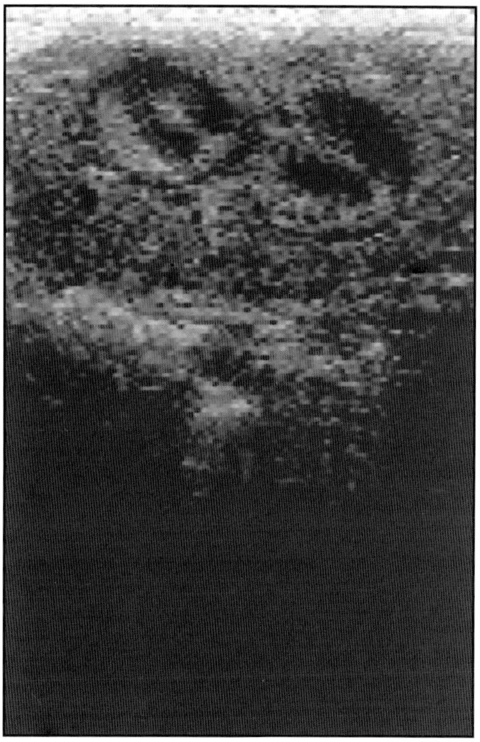

Hoofprints

Cross-sections of the rear hooves of a 200-day horse fetus and the surrounding uterine tissue

Chapter 3

SENDING AND RECEIVING

Each piezoelectric crystal in a multicrystal assembly is an individual transducer that emits sound waves and receives the returning echoes. Often, however, the term transducer is used for the entire assembly. Other terms are scanhead and probe.

The transducer functions as a remote unit that sends and receives the ultrasonic waves and echoes. The transducer is a vital, complex, and sensitive component of the ultrasound system. It is connected by a coaxial cable to the console that originates electric signals to the transducer and processes the signals from the transducer. Some consoles in veterinary ultrasound systems for large-animal reproductive work were designed for examination of humans, but the transducers were modified to allow intrarectal insertion and manipulation in large animals. For scanning the reproductive tract, the transducer is inserted into the rectum (transrectal examinations) or vagina (transvaginal examinations) or applied to the skin surface (transabdominal and transcutaneous examinations). Much attention must be given to the transducer in the selection of an ultrasound system. Important considerations in selecting transducers include frequency (e.g., 3.5, 5.0, and 7.5 MHz), ease of intrarectal insertion and manipulation, atraumatic design, durability, and quality of the image.

This chapter provides basic information on types of transducers, resolution, focusing, arrangement of the crystals and their firing format, and characteristics of the generated ultrasound beams and their relationship to the resulting image on the display screen. As cited in Chapter 2 (pg 27), the background information was obtained from literature intended for ultrasonographers in human medicine and was modified for compatibility with the transducers of ultrasound scanners being marketed for transrectal examination of the reproductive tract of animals.

Types of Transducers

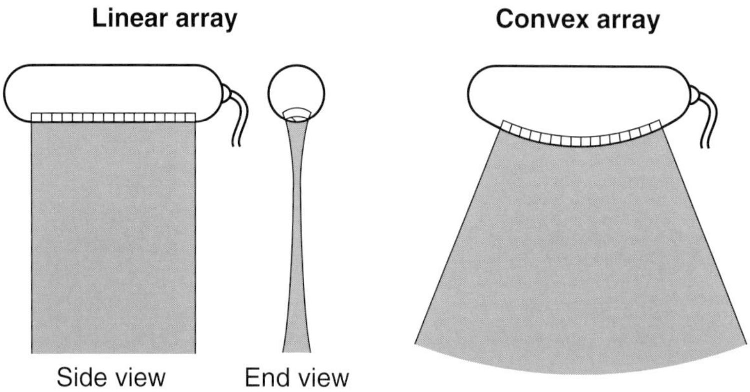

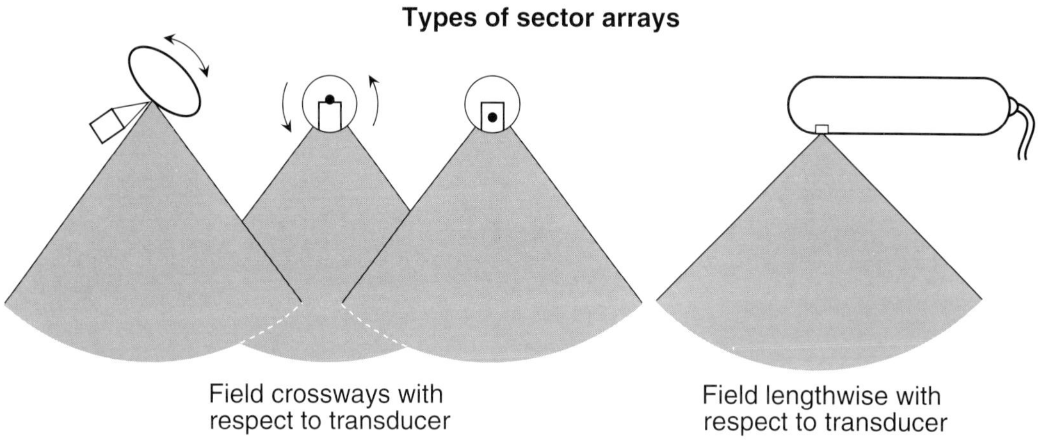

Comparison of types of transducers. Transducer refers to any device that converts energy from one form to another. Ultrasonic transducers convert electric energy into mechanical energy for production of ultrasonic waves and also convert the acoustic energy of echoes into electric energy.

Linear array refers to the side-by-side arrangement of the rectangular piezoelectric crystals along the length of the transducer. The examining field and the two-dimensional image are in the shape of a rectangle, as shown. The rectangular field of a transrectal linear-array scan is oriented longitudinally, or lengthwise, with respect to the animal. With only a few exceptions, the images shown in these volumes are from linear-array scanners. Most of the ultrasound scanners used for intrarectal examination of the reproductive tract of large animals use sequential linear-array systems.

In addition to the more common linear-array transducers, some companies market sector transducers for intrarectal use in large animals. Sector refers to the pie-shaped examining field and image. An example of an ultrasonogram from a sector scanner is shown (pg 105). In older models, the width of the pie-shaped field was oriented crossways with respect to the transducer, as shown on the lower left. Therefore, the image represented a cross-sectional sample of tissue with respect to the animal's body. Today, however, intrarectal sector transducers are being marketed in which the pie-shaped field is oriented lengthwise as shown on the lower right, similar to the orientation of the rectangular field of a linear-array probe. The width of the access to imaging is sometimes called the footprint. A large footprint (e.g., 50 mm) is characteristic of the linear format and a small footprint (e.g., 15 mm) is characteristic of the sector format. Sector transducers are especially useful for projecting beams through narrow openings, such as the space between ribs; the beams enter the tissues through a small window and then fan out. Linear-array transducers produce a real-time image by sequentially firing elements without the use of moving parts (pg 42). In sector transducers, an oscillating mirror fans the beams across the area of interest or the active portion is mechanically rotated or oscillated, as shown.

Convex or curved arrays have been introduced to produce a sector-like field with resolution similar to that of the linear array. The face of the transducer can be oriented so that the field of view encompasses tissues that lie ahead or beneath the transducer. Convex transducers are now available with some veterinary units, especially for transabdominal imaging in small animals and transvaginal ultrasound-guided placement of instruments or needles in large animals (pg 144). An example of a sonogram from a convex transducer is shown (pg 106).

Phased-array transducers are being produced in which the crystals are arranged in a linear array, but a field similar to that of a convex transducer is produced. This is accomplished by varying the electronic-delay times for each element according to the desired usage. By changing the excitation time from one frame to the next, it is possible to produce electronic steering of the wave front as opposed to physical steering *(25)*. The phased-array transducer is smaller than a linear transducer so that a sector effect is optimized; 1 to 3 cm lengths are common. Because of the complex circuitry, however, these transducers are reportedly *(25)* relatively expensive and have the potential for side-lobe degradation.

The crystals or elements of the probe are the active components for the two-way conversion of energy (pg 29). When subjected to an electric charge or to the pressure of an echo, a crystal vibrates at a natural frequency that is determined by its dimensions. Therefore, to change frequencies (e.g., 3 MHz to 5 MHz), the ultrasonographer changes transducers. The scanner switch should be turned off whenever a probe is to be connected or disconnected. For examination of the reproductive tract of animals, transducers with different frequencies can be used with a single console, because the amplifier of the console responds to a wide range of frequencies.

Much current research is being devoted to the development of plastic materials with improved acoustic properties, to replace the hard ceramic piezoelectric crystals *(172)*. Recently, switch-controlled multiple frequency transducers have become available for the animal market. Apparently, the transducer crystals can be vibrated with a sine wave, so that a desired frequency is produced within the confines of what is termed the transducer bandwidth *(135, 136)*. Improvements in manufacturing have allowed development of transducer crystals with a wide frequency spectrum. A broadband probe might provide the option of selecting frequencies, for example, of 3.5 versus 5.0 MHz or 5.0 versus 7.5 MHz. Transducers work best at their natural resonant frequency; the reduced performance resulting from the engineering required to generate selectable multiple frequencies can be at an acceptable level, however.

The selection of transducer frequencies for examination of the reproductive tract is discussed in Chapter 6 (pg 88).

Design and Firing of Linear-array Transducers

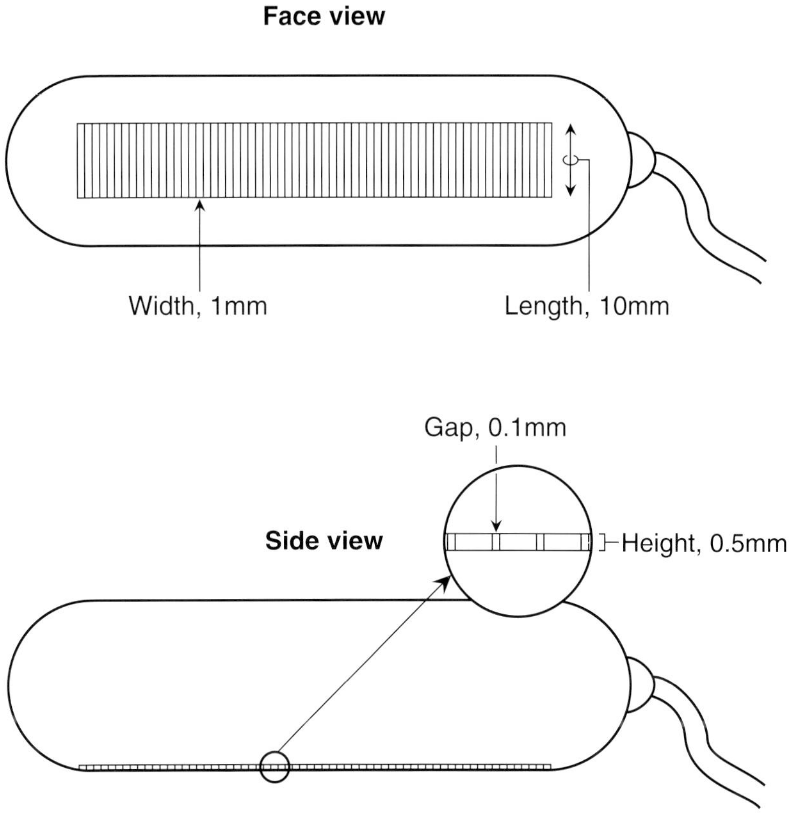

Example of arrangement of crystals in a linear-array transducer. Note the side-by-side arrangement of the array of crystals or elements in a linear orientation corresponding to the length of the transducer. Linear-array transducers consist of 60 to 120 or more elements. Some of the current models of veterinary scanners use 64 elements. In the above example, each element has face dimensions of 10 mm (length) x 1 mm (width) and a thickness of 0.5 mm. The width of an individual element corresponds to 1 or 2 wavelengths. The sound waves generated by each element are transmitted parallel to one another. The narrow element width provides closely spaced waves, thereby providing fine spatial detail of anatomical structures. Adjacent elements are separated by a narrow gap (0.1 mm), so that each crystal can vibrate independently. Usually, each element is wired independently, so that a single crystal can be fired and can receive an echo signal. On some scanners, however, a group of very fine crystals (e.g., eight per group) may be wired in common; such crystal sets are activated in unison.

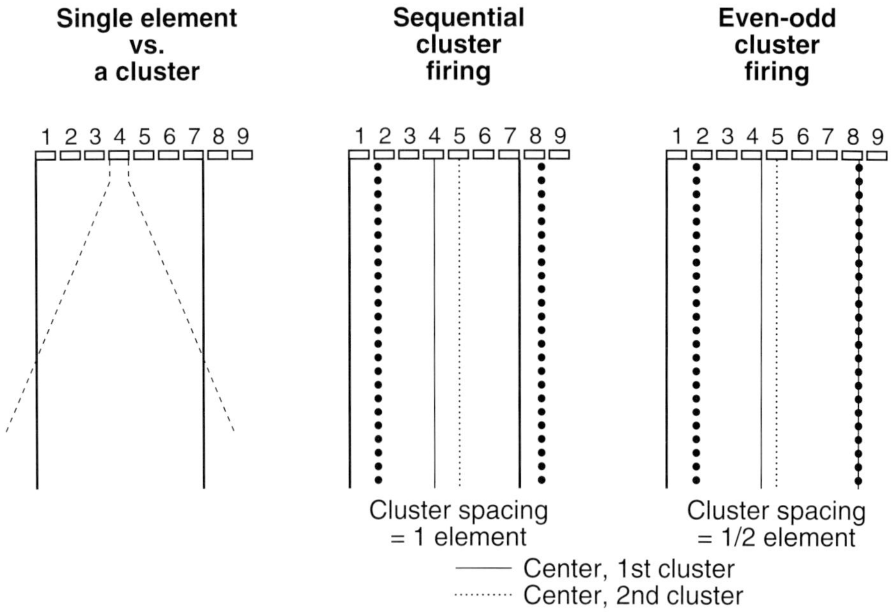

Sequential, cluster firing of the elements in linear-array transducers. Firing each element sequentially along the linear array results in unacceptable images, resulting from spreading out or diffraction of the ultrasonic beam. Diffraction is prominent when the dimensions of the source are equivalent to approximately one wavelength, and this is what occurs when a single crystal is fired. Spreading of the ultrasound beam would be undesirable because of the loss of resolution (pg 47). As shown on the left, divergence of ultrasound is more dramatic for a small source (one element) than for a large source (several elements fired in a cluster). Firing the crystals in clusters, therefore, reduces the diffraction. In addition, slightly unsynchronized firing within each cluster permits manipulation of the resulting waves to improve resolution (pg 47).

Firing clusters in sequence (e.g., crystals 1 to 7, 8 to 14, etc.) is also unacceptable. Spatially, the signals from returning echoes become assigned to the center of each cluster. Since each cluster is thus represented by a single vertical scanning line on the image display screen (pg 61), the distance between scanning lines would be far too great. These conflicting problems were solved by firing the elements in small clusters beginning at one end, and then moving the cluster format in one-element increments along the linear array. For example, a cluster of elements 1, 2, 3, 4, 5, 6, and 7 may be fired, as shown in the middle. After the cluster is activated, the same cluster is used to detect the echoes by allowing suitable time for echo reception. Then the second cluster (elements 2 to 8) is fired by moving one step down the array.

In some scanners, a system of even-odd firing is used. This system provides a finer spacing of clusters, evening out the image by increasing the number of scanning lines on the viewing screen. In the format for sequential cluster firing, described above, the cluster moves along the array in increments of one element. The effect is that the center of the cluster is moved down the array in one-element steps. In even-odd firing, a cluster is formed by firing an even number of elements (e.g., 8), followed by an odd number (e.g., 7), etc. This results in half-element spacing between the individual scanning lines that form the image on the ultrasound viewing screen, as shown, and provides for even finer spatial detail of the tissue structures. As a modification in even-odd firing, an interlacing pattern may be used wherein the even-numbered clusters are fired sequentially along the full length of the array, and then the sequence is repeated using the odd-numbered clusters.

Clearly, the design of the firing pattern has considerable influence on the quality of the resulting image. Other factors, such as the spacing of the crystals (pg 41) and housing and damping design (pg 34) profoundly affect image quality. The engineering for insulation between adjacent crystals is another factor affecting quality. Although a minimal number of elements is desirable, a transducer cannot be evaluated on the basis of number of crystals alone.

Beams and Real-time

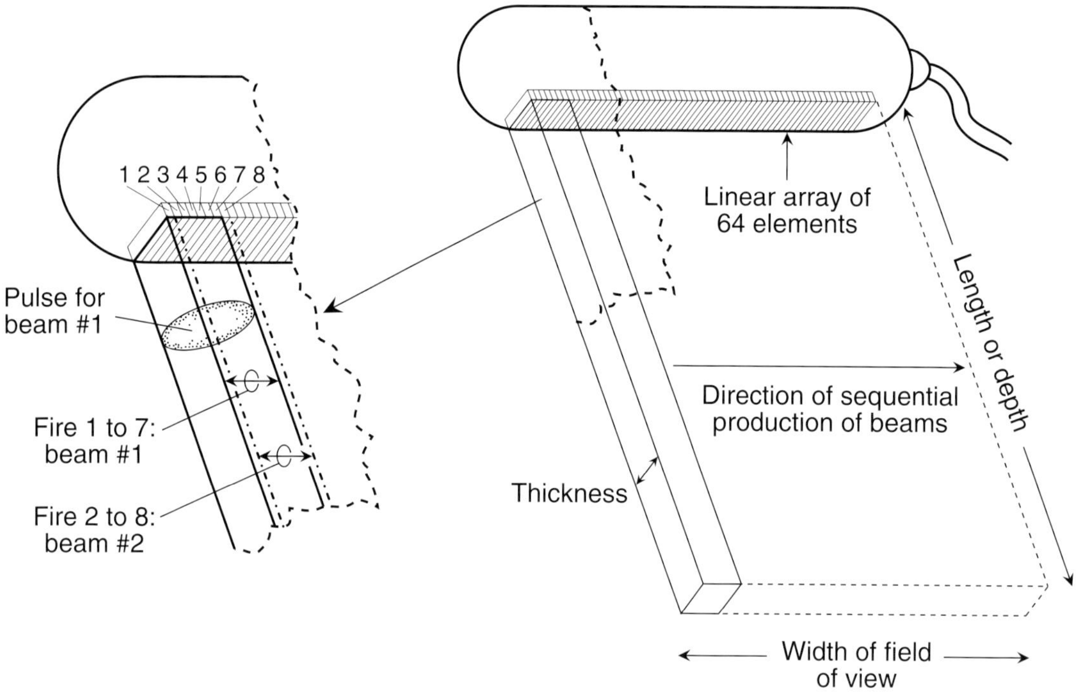

Origin and profile of unfocused linear-array ultrasound beams and the field of view resulting from a full complement of beams. The sound field resulting from firing a cluster of elements is termed a beam. A beam is shaped as though the cluster were a single large element. An echo impinging on any element in a cluster is assigned to that group of elements and to a corresponding vertical scanning line on the screen display (pg 58). It is emphasized that the beams depicted above and elsewhere are imaginary; they merely outline the three-dimensional path followed by each pulse. Only one pulse is involved in each beam, since a delay must be allowed after the firing of each pulse for the collection of echo information. Because of the high velocity of the ultrasound pulse in tissue (1.54 mm/microsecond), the echo patterns for each beam can be collected in a fraction of a millisecond.

A complete sweep of beams across all the elements in the array produces one image or frame. The use of frames permits real-time images—that is, images that move as the structures move. Detection of rapid movements requires rapid frame rates. Typical frame rates are 20 to 30 frames per second. Therefore, the movement of a beating equine embryonic heart (e.g., 150 beats/min) or the to-and-fro movement of an equine embryonic vesicle can be observed while it is occurring. Real-time is the most exciting aspect of diagnostic ultrasound. Some veterinary scanners have a frame rate, or a switch for reducing frame rate, that is too slow to detect embryonal heartbeats. Real-time not only permits the observation of movements, but also allows the operator to adjust the image while it is being observed. Fast frame rates are visually pleasing and permit moving the transducer without retaining traces of the old image. Although very high frame rates may be used for motion studies (e.g., cardiac imaging), image quality may be sacrificed because of interference with focusing and line-density capabilities. Frame rates below 20/second tend to flicker *(25)*. On the other hand, slower frame rates apparently reduce the extent of reverberation artifacts (pg 74).

The field of view encompassed by a sweep of beams extending the full length of the array of elements corresponds to the tissue region being examined. The terms width, length or depth, and thickness will be used here to define the three-dimensional area corresponding to the field of view. These terms can more easily be related to the resulting two-dimensional image on the ultrasound screen. The width of the field corresponds to the length of the row of elements and is seen as the width of the image on the screen. The length of the field corresponds to the useful or displayed depth penetrated by the beams. The remaining, smallest dimension can be called the thickness. This important dimension represents the thickness of the sampled slice of tissue; its magnitude must be imagined while viewing the image. The ultrasonographer must appreciate the magnitude of all dimensions for a given transducer in order to mentally relate the ultrasound field to the tissue mass. For simplicity, beams are depicted as rectangles in the illustration. However, focusing imparts an hourglass shape, which improves the resolution in the focal area as discussed on subsequent pages.

Beam Resolution

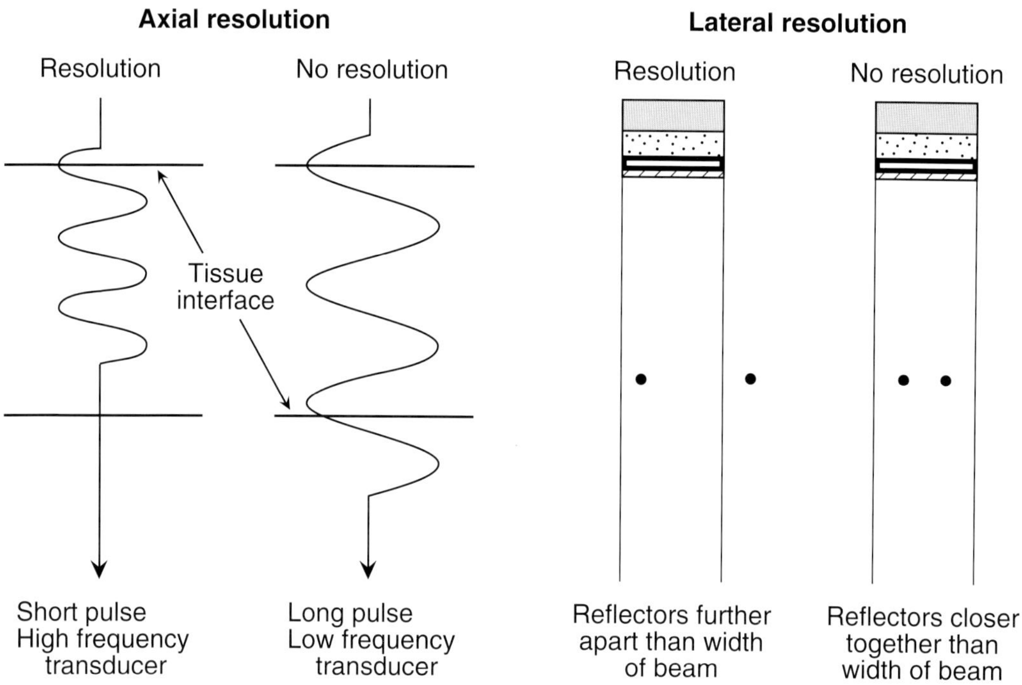

Effect of dimensions of a beam and length of a pulse on resolution. Resolution refers to the ability of an ultrasound pulse to distinguish between two closely spaced reflectors. In axial resolution, the reflectors are located along the direction of the beam. High-frequency transducers give better axial resolution, due to the relatively shorter pulses. Shorter pulses are less likely to overlap neighboring reflecting surfaces, as shown, and therefore are more likely to distinguish between them. From an engineering standpoint, axial resolution can be improved by having the transducer highly damped (pg 34) to give a short vibration time. In lateral resolution, the reflectors are located at right angles to the direction of the sound pulse. Lateral resolution can be applied to either the width or thickness of the beam. Two reflectors are resolvable when they are separated by a space greater than the beam width or thickness, whereas more closely spaced reflectors are not. When two reflectors are encompassed within the width of a beam, as shown, the two echoes arrive at the transducer simultaneously and are therefore perceived as a single echo.

Focusing

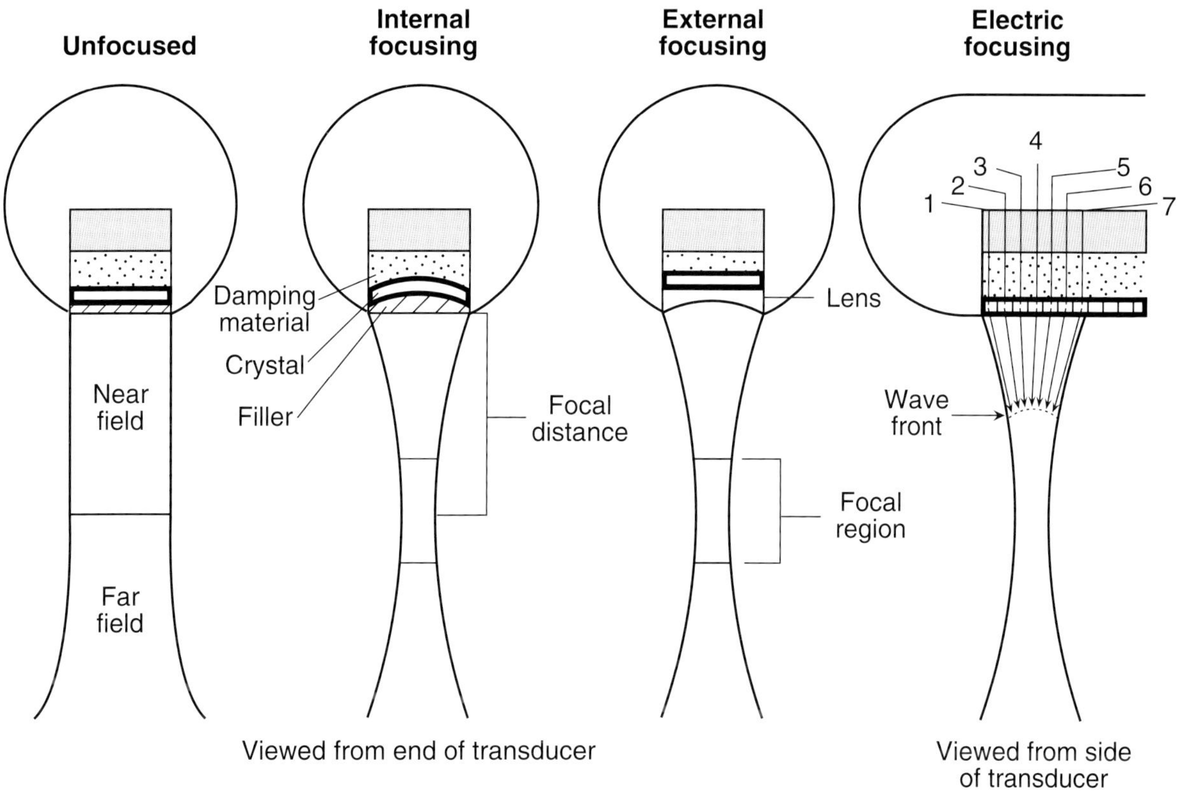

Methods of focusing. The first half of the beam nearest to the transducer source is called the near field, and the distal half is called the far field. In an unfocused beam, the junction of the near field and far field is at the point of natural divergence of the beam. The maximum lateral resolution is obtained in the near field. In the far field, the beam begins to diverge and is more likely to encompass neighboring reflectors, thereby reducing resolution (pg 46). Focusing narrows a portion of the beam profile and thereby increases the amplitude of the echoes from reflectors at a certain depth. Beams may be focused in the thickness plane to give better lateral resolution at a given depth. This is done by using curved crystals (internal focusing) or by placing an acoustic lens beneath the crystals (external focusing), as shown. By modifying the element-firing sequence, beams can also be focused in the width plane (electric focusing).

The example shown uses the firing sequence of 1-7, 2-6, 3-5, and 4. Thus, some scanners provide lateral focusing in two dimensions—the width of the beam is focused by the firing sequence and the thickness by lens or curved crystals.

It is important to select a transducer that is focused closest to the depth of interest. With higher frequency transducers, the focal region is closer to the transducer; however, there is some latitude to this rule. A 7.5 MHz transducer, for example, can be designed to have a focal region comparable to that of a 5 MHz transducer. For example, the focal distances of transducers for one veterinary scanner used for transrectal evaluation of the reproductive tract are as follows: 3.5 MHz, 70 mm; 5 MHz, 35 mm; 7.5 MHz, 20 mm. As an approximation, the effective depth for high-quality imaging is equal to twice the focal distance. A 3 MHz transducer is more suited for studying the large postpartum uterus or a large fetus by either external or intrarectal placement of the transducer. A 5 MHz transducer is best for transrectal study of the components of the reproductive tract or early conceptus. A 7.5 MHz transducer is preferred for detailed study of small structures (e.g., small ovarian follicles). As examples, the axial and lateral resolutions of focused beams, respectively, might be 1 mm and 3 mm for a 3 MHz transducer and 0.5 mm and 2 mm for a 5 MHz transducer. Axial resolution in diagnostic ultrasound is always better than lateral resolution *(25)*.

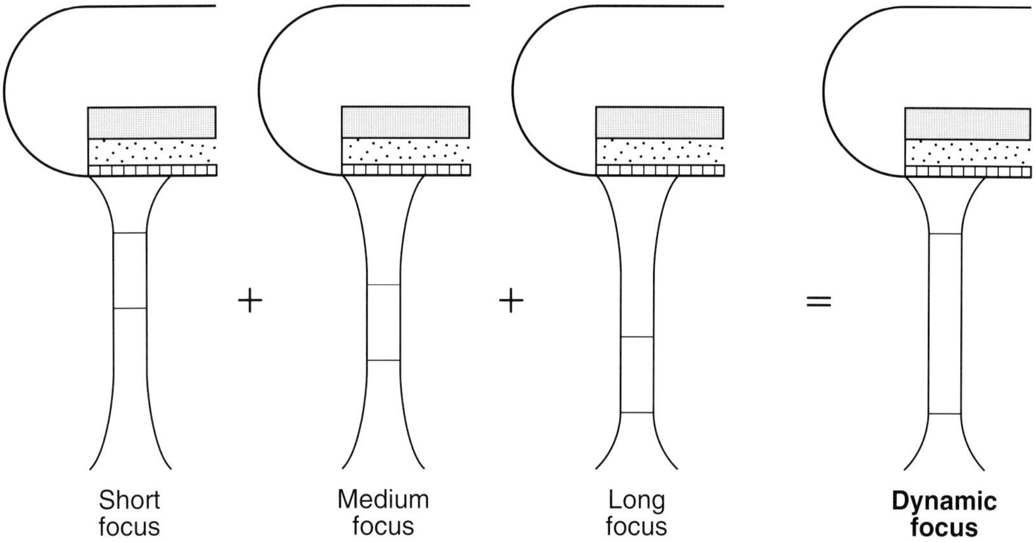

Dynamic focusing. Dynamic focusing is a form of electric focusing that results in varying focal distances rather than the fixed distance described above. This is accomplished by systematically varying the delay in the firing sequence, which in turn progressively alters the curvature of the beam front and therefore the total focal distance. Such focusing may be switch-selectable, emphasizing detail at a selected depth of interest only. In some scanners, dynamic focusing is designed to occur automatically, according to the distance traversed by the returning echoes. In switch-selectable variable focusing, the focus point can be moved through the image or multiple focal zones can be used simultaneously. However, the greater the number of selected focal zones, the slower the required frame rate. This is an important consideration when moving structures are being studied (heartbeat, embryo or fetal movements) but is less important for non-moving structures (ovary, tendon).

Production of Echo Signals

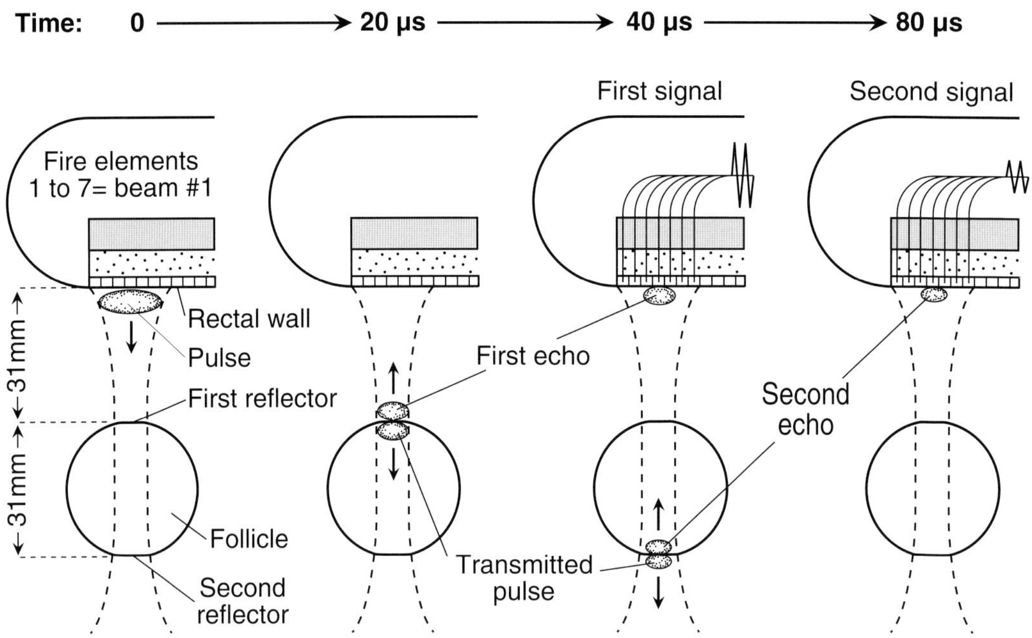

Relationships among locations of reflectors, amplitudes of echo signals, and time interval between signals. In this simplified example, a 31 mm follicle is located 31 mm from the transducer. A pulse is produced by firing the first seven elements. As the pulse travels through the tissues, it conforms to the confines of the imaginary beam. For simplicity, assume that there are only two reflectors in the field and that the speed of sound is a uniform 1.54 mm/microsecond. The pulse reaches the follicle in approximately 20 microseconds (31 mm x 1 μs/1.54 mm). When the pulse strikes the first reflector (upper surface of the follicle), part of the pulse is reflected back as the first echo, and the remainder continues on as a transmitted pulse. The first echo reaches the transducer at approximately the same time (40 μs) that the transmitted pulse reaches the far wall of the follicle, because the two distances traversed are equal (62 mm). When the echo strikes the quiescent crystals of the transducer, an electric signal is produced. The transmitted pulse is weaker than the original because of attenuation from the first reflector. Therefore, the resulting second echo and the corresponding echo signal are weaker than the first. As shown later for this example (pg 54), the disparity in amplitude between the two echo signals will be corrected by manual adjustments of the receiver. The time intervals serve to assign the proper spatial relationships for the two reflectors on the ultrasound screen (pg 55).

Chapter 4

PROCESSING

The console of ultrasound systems contains the components needed for both activating the transducer crystals at a predetermined rate and receiving and processing the returning echo signals. The console contains the controls used by the operator and the main center of attention—the viewing screen. This chapter discusses the functions of the components of the console. Consideration is given to signal amplification and the adjustment of the gain controls, the memory storage system in analog scan converters and in the more modern digital scan converters, the nature of the B-mode echo-display system, and the transfer of information in the scan converter to the echo display screen, including the relationships between scanning lines and raster lines. The presentation is a development of concepts based on published reports for medical ultrasonographers with modifications appropriate to the veterinary ultrasound scanners used for imaging the reproductive tract of animals (citations on pg 27).

Animal ultrasound scanners developed before 1983 used the analog scan converter, in which an electron beam is deflected by signals onto a plate that contains addresses corresponding to an X (horizontal) and Y (vertical) axis; such scanners were durable and some are still in use. This was accomplished by measuring the amplitude of the electric charge at a given XY location; the charge then was assigned a particular level of gray on the display screen. The analog converter is less stable and less resistant to electronic noise, because the quantitative representations of signal amplitude and time involve a continuum. Another disadvantage of the analog system is that the resulting images are not directly adaptable to videotaping and other manipulative procedures. However, excellent still photographs can be prepared from images produced by the analog system. Many of the ultrasonograms (photographs of images from an ultrasound scanner) in this text were made with an analog system (e.g., pg 10, pg 60, pg 67).

Components of a Scanner

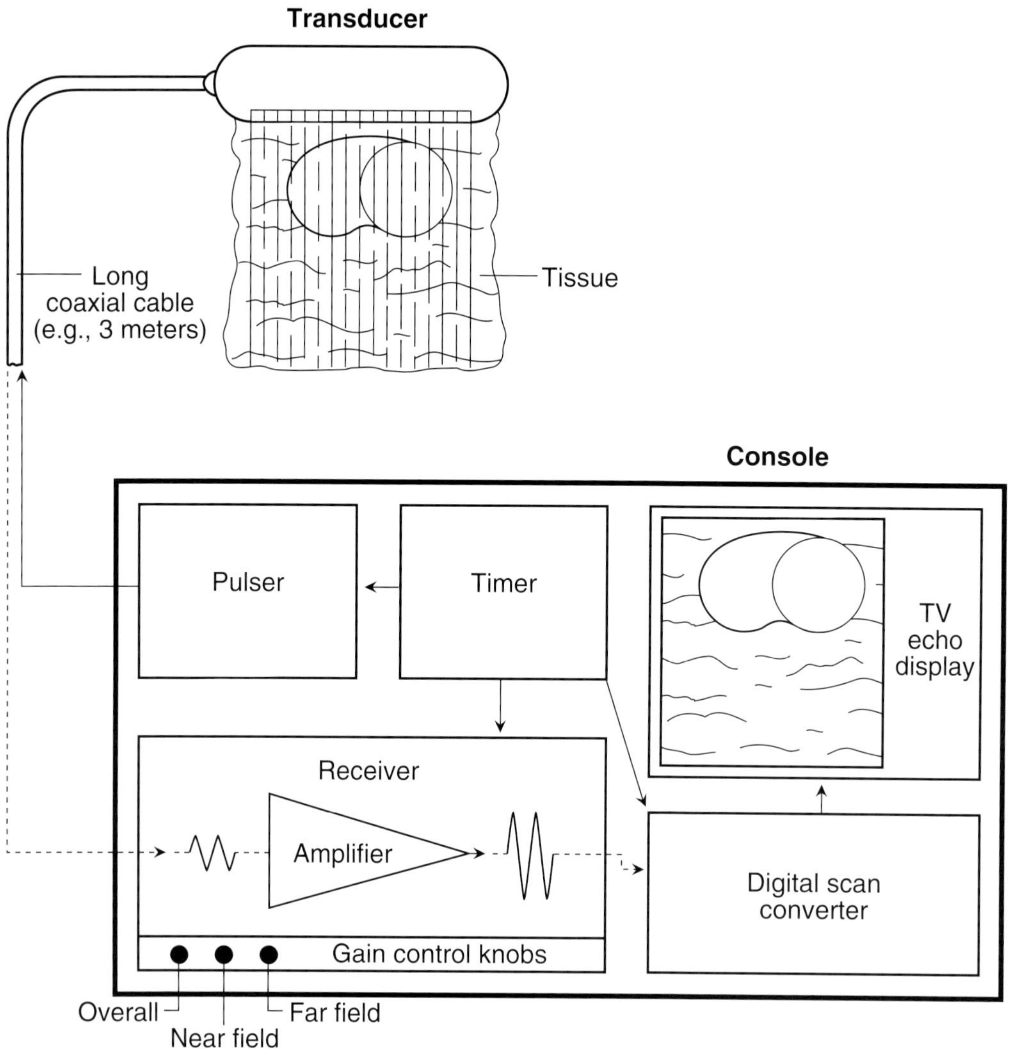

Components of a linear-array ultrasound scanner. Modern ultrasound scanners use digital, rather than analog, scan converters. The pulser, or transmitter, provides electric signals at a predetermined rate for driving the piezoelectric crystals of the transducer. The pulsating rate is such that the display of echo signals on the screen appears to be continuous. The pulse-echo cycle begins with two simultaneous events: 1) A sharp electric pulse is sent from the pulser to the transducer, and 2) An electron beam in the display cathode ray tube (pg 57) begins to move from a location that represents the transducer-tissue contact surface. Tissue echoes that leave the transducer are very small, in the millivolt and microvolt range. The echoes are initially processed by the receiver, where the echo signal is amplified and compensation is made for loss of intensity due to attenuation. This initial handling of the signals occurs before storage in the scan converter and is called preprocessing. The degree of amplification is called gain and is comparable to volume in the control of audible sound. The concept of gain must be thoroughly understood because proper adjustment of the gain knobs is one of the most important variables under the continuous control of the veterinary ultrasonographer.

The scan converter stores the amplified signals and shows the resulting information on an echo display screen. The scan converter utilizes the digital system that is used in personal computers. Since the scan information is in digital form, the output can be readily manipulated (e.g., videotaping, photographic processing, highlighting). The converter functions like the memory of a computer by recording the strength of each echo signal at an address that corresponds to the location of the echo source. The television display screen uses a similar address system, so that the addresses and the accompanying code for level of gray are read from the converter to the corresponding address on the television screen. The digital scan converter is also the major synchronizer in the system; the timing of events within the converter involves regulating the transducer scanning rate on one side and the television format on the other. Storage of the data representing signals provides the opportunity not only to see the completed image but also to manipulate the image into a preferred form. A manipulation done after the data are stored is called postprocessing; that is, the echo signals are manipulated on transfer from the scan converter to the display screen *(106)*. Postprocessing allows the operator to change the visual contrast among the echo signals that occur during scanning or on a frozen image. In most modern scanners, the preprocessing is fixed, but postprocessing can be used to change the gray-scale characteristics on the screen. Postprocessing includes automatic electronic smoothing of the image and operator-controlled positioning of calipers on the image to measure distances.

Signal Amplification

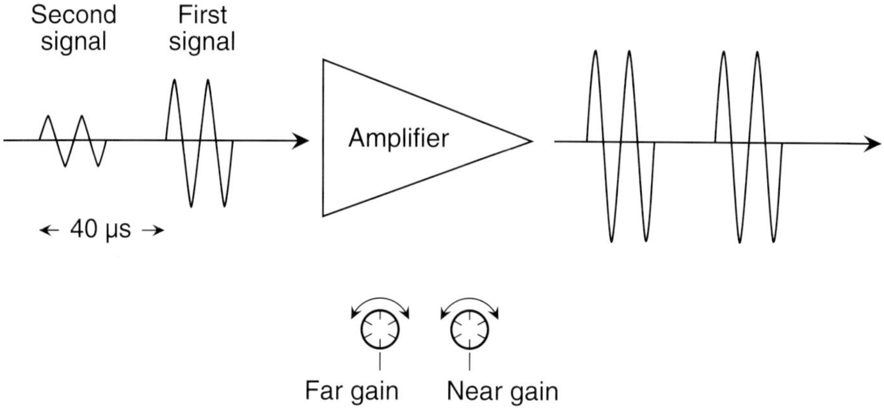

Adjustment of gain controls to equalize signal amplitude. The depicted signals are 40 microseconds apart, corresponding to reflectors 31 mm and 62 mm from the transducer, as shown previously (pg 50). Although the echogenicity of the two reflectors was similar, the amplitude of the second signal is weaker because of attenuation resulting from the interaction between the pulse and the first reflector. The amplifier greatly increases the strength of both signals in preparation for further processing. Because the two signals represent similar reflectors, the gain controls are manually adjusted, as shown, so that the amplified signals are of similar strength. This adjustment is made while viewing the resulting echoes on the image display. Proper adjustment of the gain controls is crucial in building a balanced and pleasing image.

On some scanners, controls are provided for time gain compensation (TGC) or depth gain compensation (DGC). These controls allow the operator to compensate for attenuation by equalizing the echoes coming from different tissue depths; echo signals from distant reflectors are amplified more by the control system than are those from close reflectors. On most scanners used for animal sonography, near gain, far gain, and overall gain controls are provided for the near field, far field, and the overall image, respectively. Proper balancing of the controls is needed to provide maximum clarity at various depths and to minimize artifactual responses; adjustment is discussed elsewhere (pg 97). The near-gain setting affects primarily the amplification in the first few centimeters and is needed especially to reduce the large-amplitude echoes near the transducer. The far-gain control is less important when viewing reproductive tract tissues that are close to the transducer. Far gain is more important when visualizing large or distant structures (e.g., fetus, postpartum uterus).

Digital Scan Converter

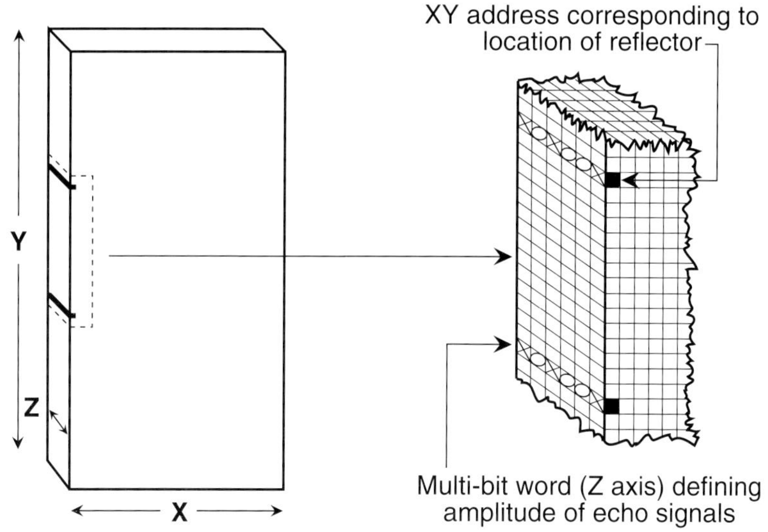

Memory storage system in digital scan converters. The scan converter memory stores the appropriate information for location of the reflector and amplitude of the echo. The digital system uses discrete circuits known as bits. "Bit" is an abbreviation for binary digit; each bit represents one of two levels of a quantity. A string of bits forms a multibit word. The number of discrete values represented by various numbers of bits in a word is as follows: 2 bits, 4 levels; 4 bits, 16 levels; 5 bits, 32 levels; 6 bits, 64 levels. Therefore, a six-bit word can represent up to 64 shades of gray, according to the amplitude of the incoming echo signal. Most current instruments in the animal market use words of six bits (64 echo levels) to represent the gray-scale value at each address. If too few shades are used (e.g., 16) the image has too much contrast, whereas too many shades (e.g., 256) may give too little contrast. The capacity of the memory storage system of scanners can be judged on the basis of the number of bits used. The data are stored in computer chips mounted on circuit boards. Mathematically, but not physically, the organization of the memory for entry and subsequent reading of echo data can be illustrated, as shown. The example relates to the previously described tissue reflectors located 31 and 62 mm from the transducer (pg 50). Addresses are represented by the XY axes and echo amplitude by the Z axis (multi-bit word). Each multi-bit word is shown consisting of six bits, which describe, according to echo intensity, the shade of gray for each memory location. In this example, the amplitude of the two processed signals was similar, as a result of manual adjustments of the gain control knobs (pg 54)

B-Mode Display

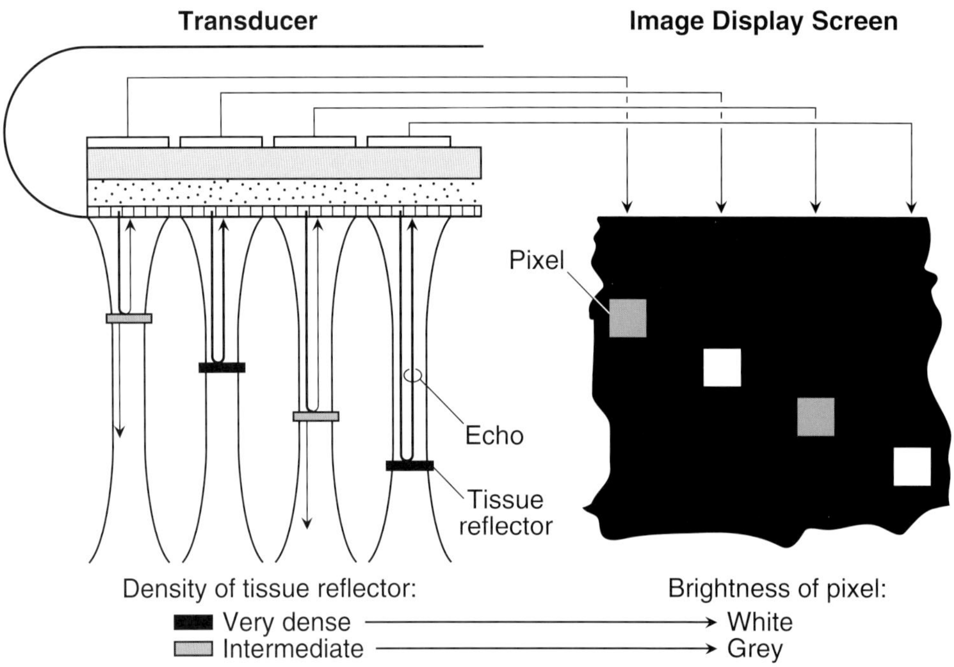

B-mode echo-display system. The ultrasound scanners described in this text use sequential linear-array transducers or sector transducers (pg 38), real-time imaging (pg 44), and B-mode echo display. The term B-mode refers to brightness modulation of the dots, or pixels, on the echo display screen. Each pixel or picture element corresponds to a location in the scan converter memory, that in turn corresponds to the location of a tissue reflector. Veterinary scan converters, for example, may use a memory size that is 114 units wide and 450 units high (51,300 pixels). The distance from the top of the image to the pixel represents the distance from transducer to tissue reflector, as shown. The brightness of a pixel corresponds to the amplitude of that individual echo signal. Brightness is represented by shades of gray extending from white (very bright or highly echogenic) to black (no discernible echo; anechoic or nonechogenic). For clarity, the size of the pixels is greatly exaggerated in the illustration. Tissue reflectors that are very dense are shown reflecting all of the sound pulse, resulting in white pixels. Reflectors of intermediate density are shown returning only a portion of the pulse, resulting in gray pixels. The terms hypoechogenic (hypoechoic), hyperechogenic (hyperechoic), and isoechogenic (isoechoic) are sometimes used to describe low, high, and uniform intensities of echogenicity, respectively. The parenthetical form of the terms appears to be increasing in usage.

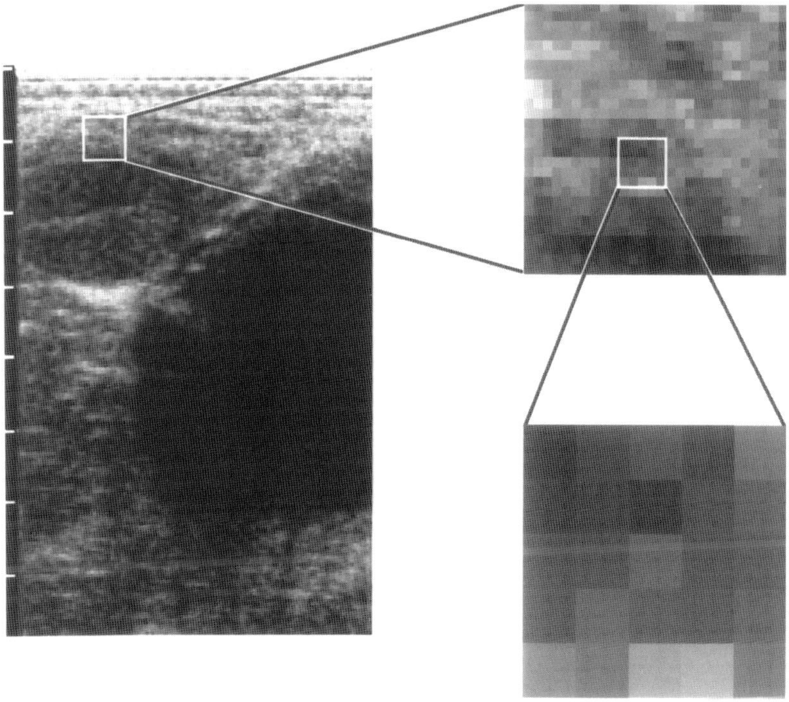

Picture elements. The sonogram shows an image of a bovine ovary (upper left) with a corpus luteum. A square (6 x 6 mm) has been placed on the ovarian stroma with the lower side at the upper edge of the corpus luteum. The selected area has been enlarged sixfold so that the picture elements or pixels are clearly visible. An area of the enlargement has been further enlarged so that the individual pixels are even more distinct. The image has approximately 48 pixels/cm, whereas the first enlarged area has approximately 8 pixels/cm and the second enlargement has 1.4 pixels/cm. Scanners in which individual pixels can be detected on the ultrasound screen without magnification are unsatisfactory. In the animal market in the 1980s, several ultrasound companies promoted and sold scanners that were so pixelated that individual picture elements were visible on the scanner screen.

Display Screen

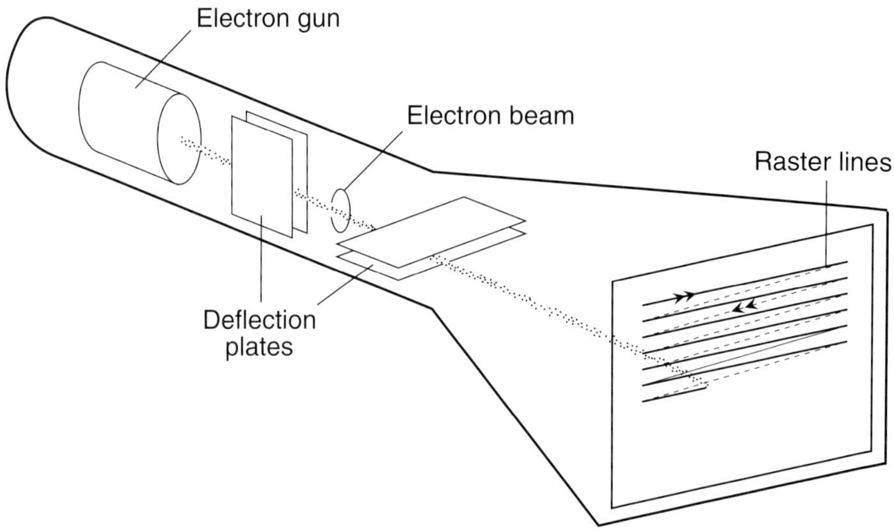

Transfer of the information in the scan converter to the echo-display screen. Electrons ("cathode rays") are produced by heating a filament in the electron gun of an oscilloscope. The cathode ray tube provides a vacuum for free passage of the electrons toward a positively charged screen. The electrons are focused into a well-defined electron beam. The beam strikes the phosphor in the screen, causing it to emit light. The beam is directed across the screen by electric signals applied to the deflection plates. This system is the same as that used in television sets.

The pattern of movement of the electron beam across the viewing screen is called a raster scan. The scan pattern begins in the upper left corner of the screen, moves steadily across, snaps back, and then begins another line, as shown. The result is a pattern of beam movement over the screen that forms a sweep or set of horizontal raster lines. In contrast to a simple oscilloscope display, the electron-beam scanning arrangement of most ultrasound viewing screens involves two sets of raster lines (sweeps) across the screen to produce an image frame. In a 450-line screen, each sweep results in the filling of 225 lines—every other one. The raster scan then jumps to the top of the screen and starts another sweep, which fills in the remaining lines. Each sweep takes 1/60th of a second and both sweeps require 1/30th of a second. Therefore, 30 complete frames are produced in one second, each frame being a composite of the two sweeps. This arrangement reduces flicker on the screen. The rapid frame rate is needed for the real-time aspect of modern diagnostic ultrasonography.

Scanning Lines

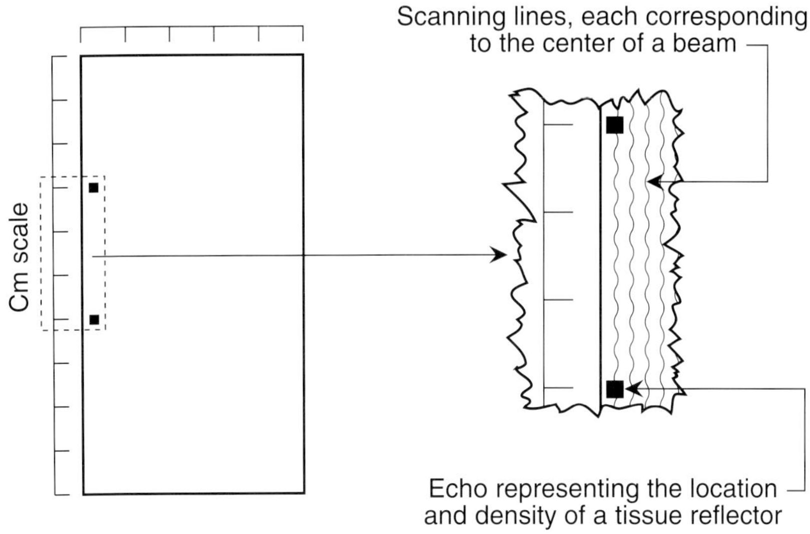

Scanning lines and the placement of echo data on the viewing screen. This example of the placement of the echo information onto the viewing screen corresponds with the tissue reflectors described earlier. For an overview of the simplified example extending from generation of an ultrasound pulse to the appearance of an echo on the screen, review the figures on the following pages in sequence: events at the transducer and tissue (pg 50); echo signal amplification (pg 54); storage of location and intensity data in the scan converter (pg 55); formation of the image (this page). Each vertical scanning line on the TV image records the information gathered by the corresponding transducer beam. Note that the echo display for each tissue reflector is placed in the appropriate location (first scanning line, 31 and 62 mm from rectal wall).

As the raster lines move across the screen, the electron beam turns on and off and thereby produces the vertical scanning lines. Therefore, each point at which a raster line crosses a scanning line represents one pixel. The intensity of the electric signals originating from the memory of the scan converter (pg 53) provides the appropriate information for the intensity (gray-scale level) of the oscilloscope's electron beam for each pixel. Thus, the information stored at each address of the converter is transferred to each pixel of the viewing screen as the sweeping beam of electrons passes over the appropriate pixel. Digital systems are very fast; recording into the memory, modifying data, and transferring data to the screen can all be done without one process interfering with the others.

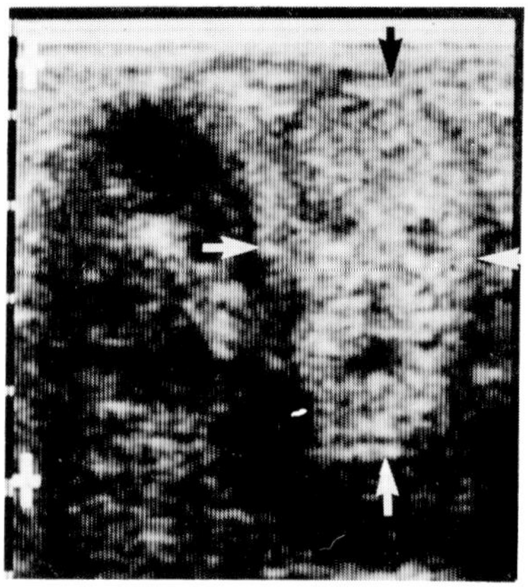

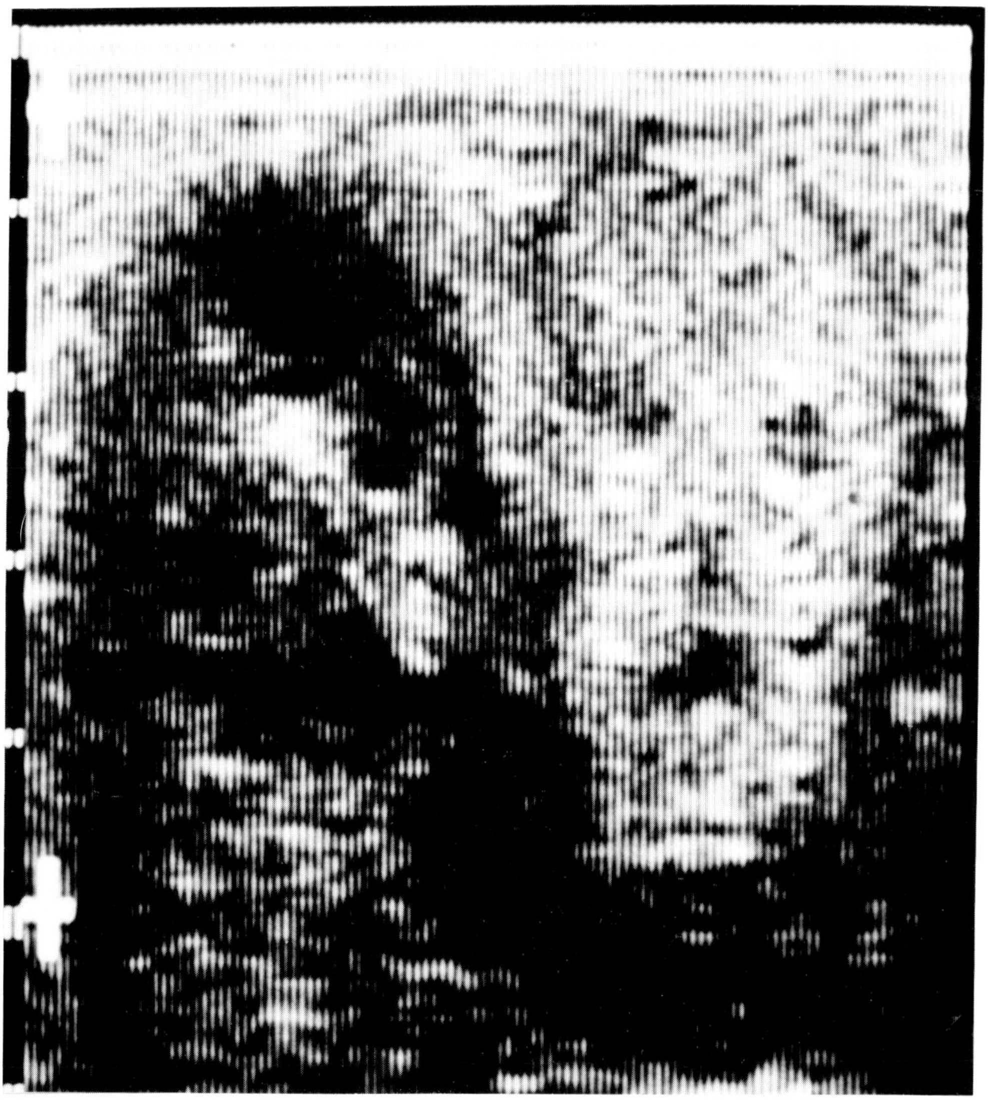

Example of scanning lines. The image of an equine corpus luteum is delineated by arrows in the smaller ultrasonogram. The scale marks are in centimeters. This luteal image, which has the appearance of a ghostly face, was seen by R. A. Pierson during thesis research on the ultrasonic anatomy of the luteal glands. Note that the scanning lines are much more obvious in the enlarged ultrasonogram. There are 114 scanning lines over the width of the image. The width of the field of view encompassing the 114 lines is 56 mm. This scanner used 64 elements. Firing consisted of the even-odd format, and therefore the scanning lines are separated by half-element spacings (pg 43). The number is less than 128 (half-element spacing for 64 elements) because there is a mathematical loss of some elements on each end of the transducer; each scanning line conforms to the center of each fired cluster of elements (pg 42).

A comparison between the small and large images demonstrates that scanning lines become more obvious when an ultrasonogram is enlarged, if the distance from the sonogram to eyes is held constant. Note, however, that the scanning lines in the enlargement begin to disappear as the distance from sonogram to eyes is increased. For this reason, if the scanning lines on a given scanner are bold and considered unpleasant, increasing the distance from screen to eyes may be more acceptable. This same principle applies to scanners with zoom or magnification controls. The scanning lines may be more obvious upon magnification, unless the distance from observer to screen is increased. At the optimal distance, the eye tends to provide a smoother picture. The sonograms from some scanners using digital scan converters do not show distinct scanning lines. Such scanners may use an electronic system to average the intensities between adjacent lines, thereby tending to fill in the spaces between lines. The image, therefore, has a smoother appearance than the one shown in this figure. The quality of engineering in the display system is a source of variation in image quality. Part of the smoothness of the digital television image comes from the use of very small pixels. Some scanners sold in the veterinary market, especially in the 1980s, were undesirable because large pixels gave the image a checkered appearance.

In some portable scanners (e.g., Aloka 210), the conventional format of vertical scanning lines and horizontal raster lines is rotated 90 degrees, so that the scanning lines are horizontal and the raster lines are vertical. When videotapes prepared from such scanners are played back on the scanner monitor, they are properly oriented. However, when shown on a television viewing screen with the conventional format, the image is oriented on its side. More recent models (e.g., Aloka 500) have eliminated this problem.

The Net Result

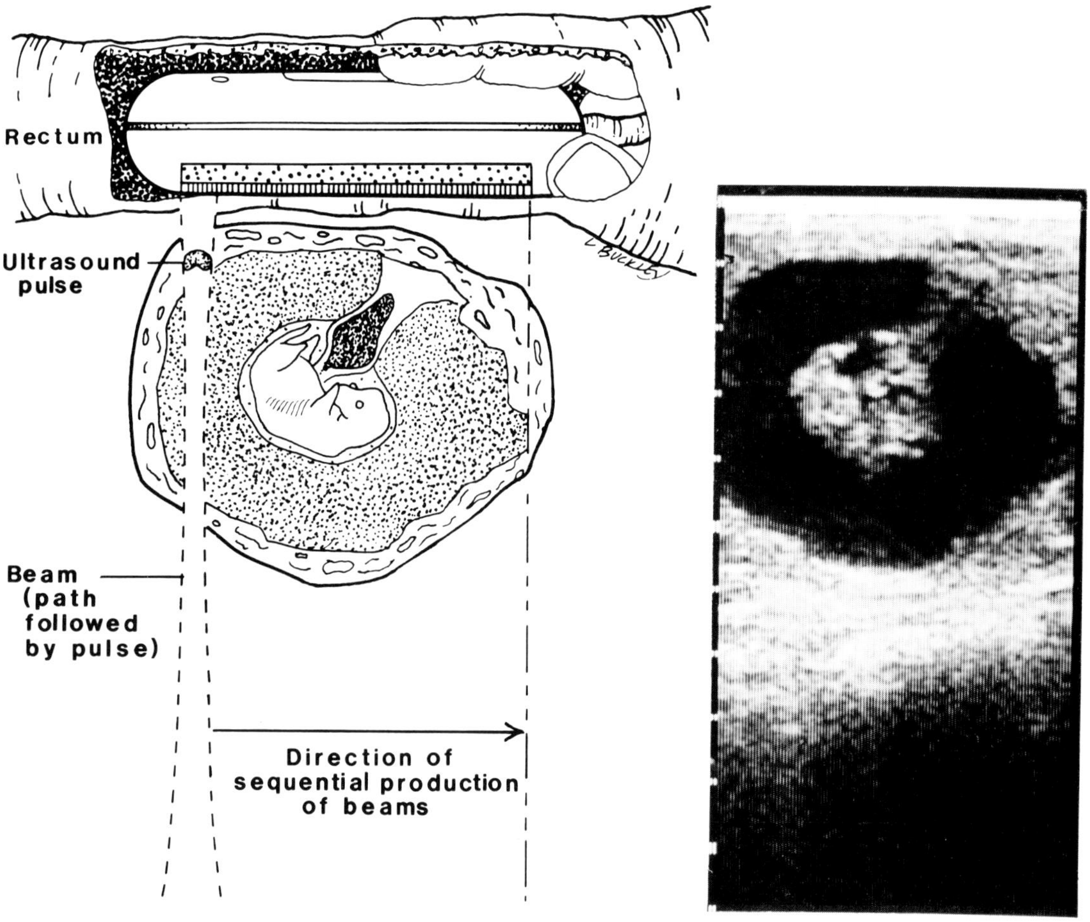

Development of an image of a 45-day equine fetus. A 64-element linear-array transducer is held in the rectum over a uterine horn. An ultrasound pulse is generated by firing a cluster of elements. The resulting pulse follows the confines of the imaginary focused beam, and echo signals are returned to the same elements. After completion of echo-gathering data, the cluster moves down the array and a second pulse is fired, producing a second beam. This sequential, segmental firing of clusters of elements moves along the array, completing 30 passes per second. The resulting echo signals are processed, resulting in a displayed image. Each picture element (pixel) corresponds to a location of a tissue reflector, and the brightness of each pixel corresponds to the density (echo-producing ability) of the tissue reflector. The information from each beam is displayed by a corresponding scanning line on the screen. The image represents a thin, two-dimensional slice through the tissue. Slowly moving the transducer produces sequential slices, which are displayed as images corresponding to the orientation of the transducer. Thus, a real-time mental image of the three-dimensional aspects of the moving fetus is obtained.

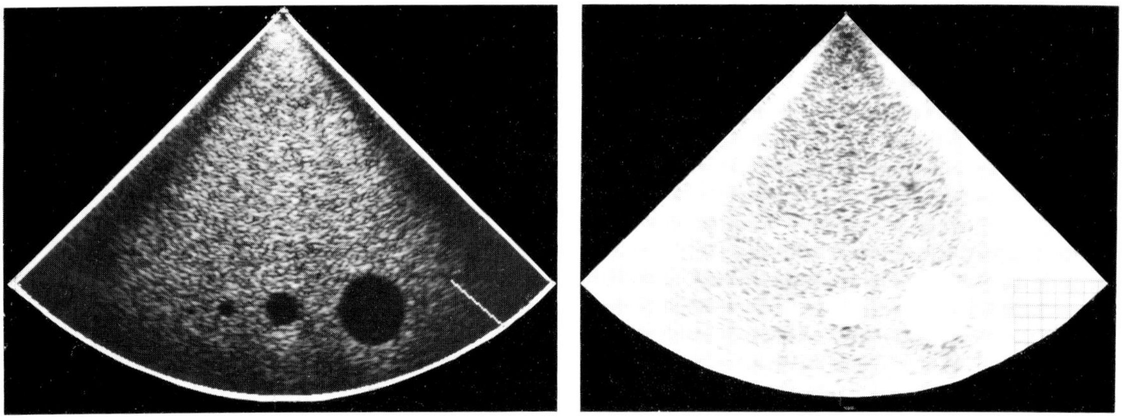

Images from a sector scanner showing two formats. The specimen is an ultrasonic phantom containing fluid-filled objects (largest=20 mm) at a depth of 80 mm. The image on the left is in the white-on-black format used on current linear-array and sector scanners for examination of the reproductive tract of animals. However, some ultrasonographers in human medicine prefer the reverse black-on-white format shown on the right; the background is white and the brightest pixels are black. Some scanners are equipped with a video inverse switch so either format can be chosen. An ultrasonographer who has worked with only one format may have difficulty when first presented with the opposite format. Apparently, white-on-black provides better boundary information and black-on-white provides better textural information. In the above images, the outlines of the non-echogenic, fluid-filled spheres seem more distinct on the white-on-black image (left), whereas the ultrasonic texture of the remaining simulated tissue seems more pronounced on the black-on-white image (right). Sometimes the availability of both formats aids in the interpretation of echoes from a suspicious area. It is easier for a beginner to relate to the white on-black format because of familiarity with light rays. Thus, an intense reflection of either light or an ultrasound echo (as seen on the image) is a bright spot, and a shadow is a black area behind a light barrier or beneath a dense ultrasound reflector (e.g., bone).

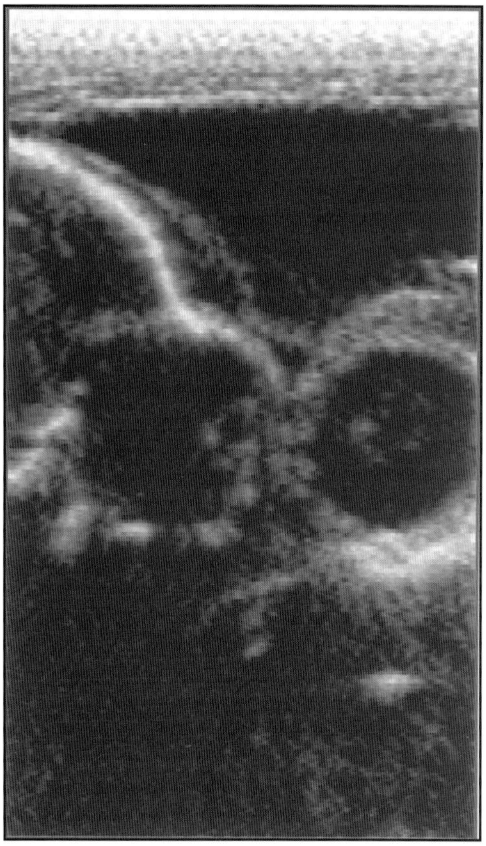

Eye to Eye

One eye of each member of a 140-day equine fetal twin set.

Chapter 5

INTERPRETING

Interpreting ultrasound images is one of those disciplines for which learning is never complete. Even after much experience, a sonographer may see an image formation that had not been noticed before—only to find that thereafter the formation is disconcertingly common and obvious. Proper interpretation of the echoes on an ultrasound screen requires knowledge of the relationships between tissues and echoes and the ability to differentiate between factual and artifactual responses. This chapter will describe the two types of factual reflections (specular and nonspecular), which are presented as echoes on the screen, and the associations between them and tissue structure.

Ultrasonic imaging represents an interaction between the complexity of the scanner and the complexity of the tissues. Certain tissue formations cause sound waves to bend (refract), bounce back and forth or re-echo (reverberate), become weakened (attenuated), or entirely blocked. As a result, artifactual distortions appear on the ultrasound image and can be mistaken for normal or pathological structures or changes. Some ultrasonographers seemingly develop the ability to subconsciously disregard artifacts; this may be a mistake because artifacts also provide information on tissue structure and on improper gain settings. Artifacts are especially common during imaging of the reproductive tract because of the many pockets of bowel gas, fluid-filled structures, and pelvic and fetal bone. This chapter will describe the nature and origin of the artifacts common in this area, including shadowing, enhancement, reverberation, and beam-width artifacts.

Artifactual echoes and the nature of the ultrasound technology can lead to befuddlement in the interpretation process—so much so, that individuals who are in the forefront of evaluating and using ultrasound scanners for research and clinical purposes must accept the risk that they may describe an interesting biological structure that others may later show was an artifact or the natural result of the imaging technology. In this regard, in the early 1980s ultrasonograms were published in which the specular echo on an image of an embryonic vesicle was erroneously labeled the embryonic disc. Such misinterpretations are easily made. However, knowledge of the nature and origin of factual and artifactual echoes should minimize the occurrence of such misinterpretations.

Specular Reflections

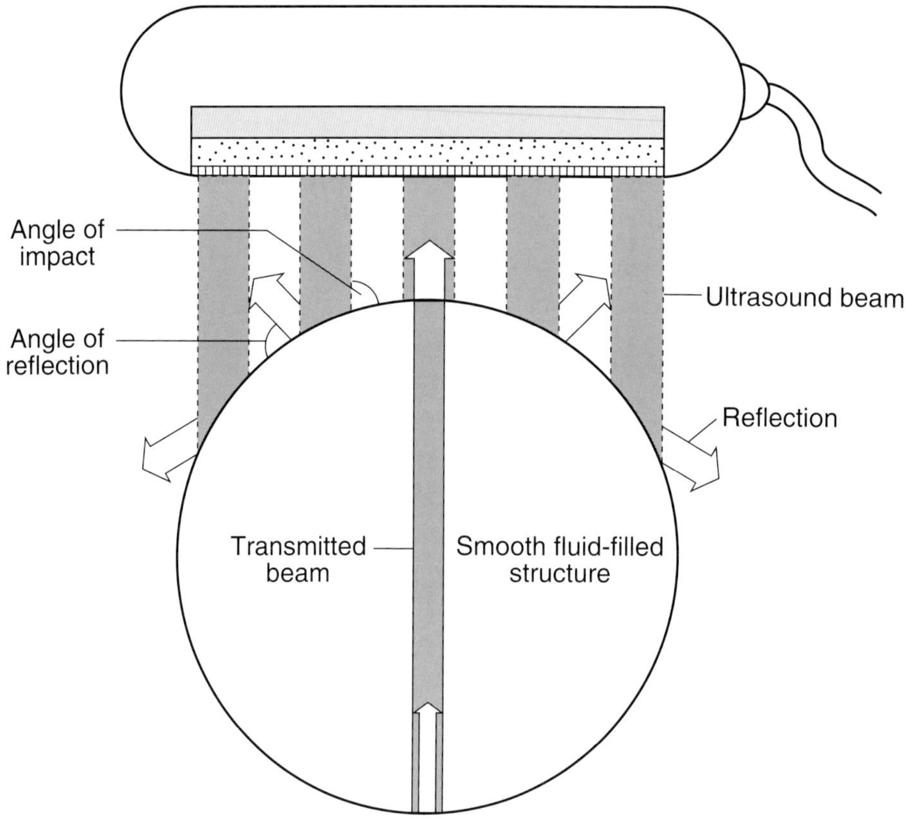

Angle of impact of a sound beam and specular reflections. A specular reflection results when a beam strikes an interface that is smooth, wider than the beam, and parallel to the transducer. Usually only a small portion of the pulse that strikes such an interface is reflected. The major portion of the pulse continues past the interface as a transmitted pulse or beam, as shown. If the wall on the opposite side of an encapsulated, fluid-filled structure is smooth, the opposite wall also will act as a specular reflector. Only a pulse that strikes a specular reflector at approximately a right angle will be recorded as an echo on the screen. Therefore, the intensity of the echo is determined not only by the difference in acoustic impedance between the two tissues making up the interface, but also by the angle of incidence (angle of impact). Pulses that strike the interface at other than a right angle are reflected at an equal angle into the tissue and the interface will not be detected; the orientation of the transducer must be changed. Specular reflections are very common in images of the reproductive tract. The smooth surface of the external uterus, endometrial folds, embryonic vesicles, and uterine cysts are all examples of prominent specular reflectors.

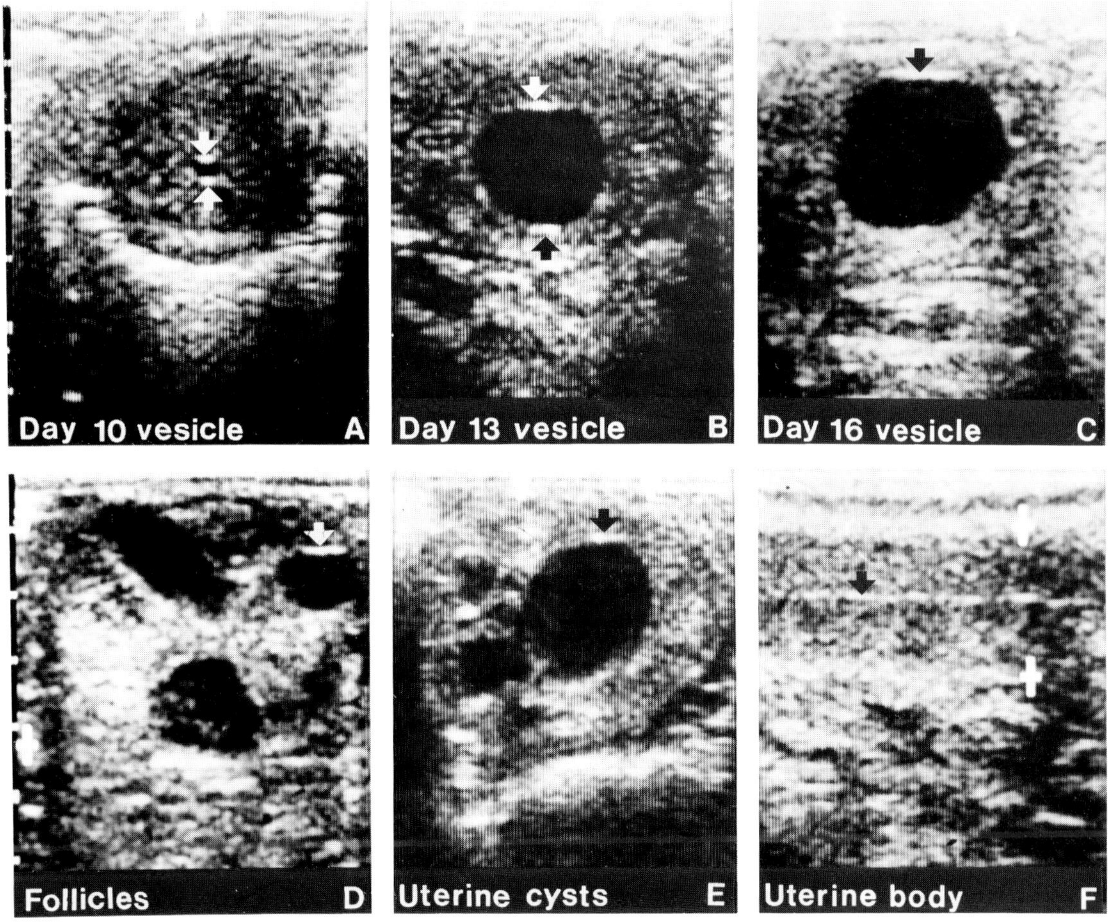

Examples of specular echoes from the reproductive tracts of mares. The echoes (arrows) are bright or hyperechogenic and parallel to the surface of the transducer (upper edge of image). The echoes can be seen both on the upper and lower surfaces of the Day-10 and Day-13 embryonic vesicles (A, B). A specular echo is not discernible on the bottom of the Day-16 embryonic vesicle (C), probably because the surface is not smooth or because the echo is obscured by the high degree of echogenicity in the soft tissue beneath the vesicle. The echogenicity beneath the vesicle results from enhancement and is discussed elsewhere (pg 71). Specular echoes are also seen on the surface of the images of ovarian follicles (D). Sometimes the transducer must be rotated slightly to demonstrate a specular reflection from a follicle; the orientation of the transducer and surface of the follicle must be compatible, as shown in the diagram (pg 66). The specular echo on the large compartment of the uterine cystic complex (E) is attributable to the smooth surface of a dome-like fluid-filled projection into the uterine lumen. Frequently, the uterine lumen is seen as a bright echogenic line when the uterus is viewed longitudinally (F), presumably resulting from specular reflections from the surface of uterine folds.

Nonspecular Reflections

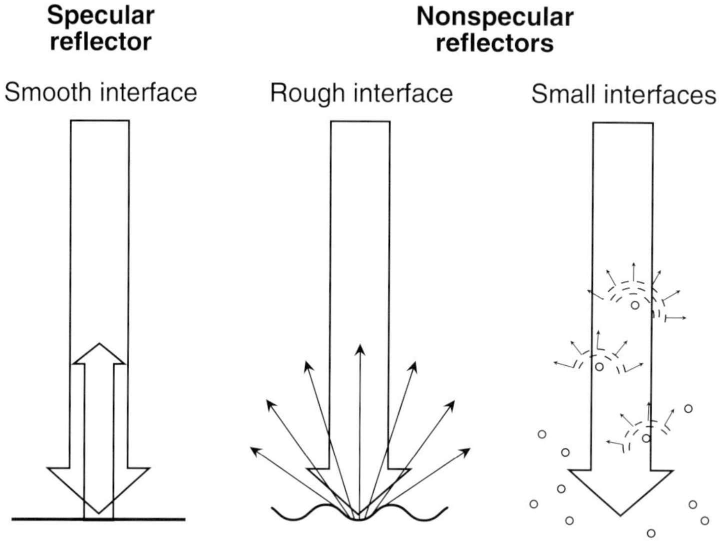

Comparison of the origins of specular and nonspecular echoes. Nonspecular, scattered, or diffuse reflections originate when a pulse strikes a rough interface or one that is narrower than the pulse. In contrast to specular reflectors, echo amplitude for nonspecular reflectors is not dependent on beam angle. Ultrasound pulses in the focal zone have dimensions of 2 or 3 mm. Interfaces smaller than these approximate figures therefore give rise to nonspecular reflections. When the ultrasound pulse enters a heterogeneous medium or strikes a rough surface, the effective interfaces are narrower than the beam, and scatter of echoes occurs, as shown. Scatter is defined as the redirection of sound in many directions. A small portion of the scattered echoes are directed back toward the sound source, and these are referred to as backscatter. The amplitude of the echoes reaching the transducer from a scatterer is very low (e.g., 1/100 of the amplitude of a specular echo). Since the pulse encounters many scatterers simultaneously, many echoes are generated at once. Some of these may arrive at the transducer at one time and may either reinforce or interfere with others. The net result is a displayed pattern, texture, or speckling that helps to identify a given tissue or to distinguish one tissue from another (e.g., corpus luteum versus surrounding stroma). This delineation may be possible even in the absence of an intervening capsule acting as a specular reflector. Gray-scale imaging fully utilizes the scatter phenomenon of nonspecular or diffuse reflections. It should be appreciated that the bright and dark regions of a speckled area do not necessarily correspond to physical tissue structures. Instead, the speckled pattern is an interference pattern that nevertheless may be representative of an organ or tissue and is referred to as the tissue's <u>echotexture</u>. Because the echo amplitude is independent of beam angle (unlike specular reflectors), the shade of gray (echo amplitude) for a given cellular tissue is more nearly constant regardless of transducer orientation. Scatter causes the vast majority of diagnostic echoes in cellular organs.

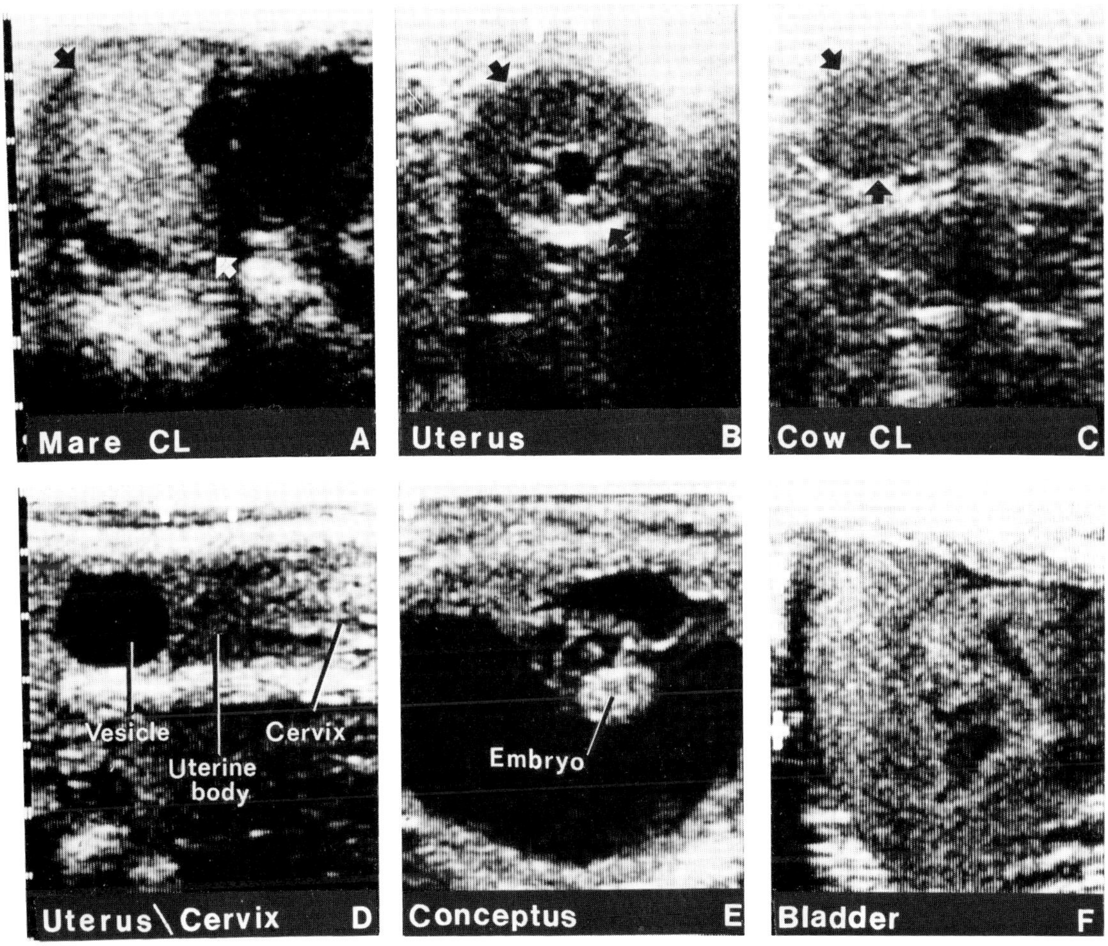

Examples of nonspecular echoes from mares (A, B, D, E, F) and a cow (C). CL=corpus luteum. Compare the ultrasonic echotextures of the indicated tissues. Note the marked differences in echotexture between the uterine body and the denser cervix (D). The urinary bladder (F) of horses normally contains particles large enough to act as diffuse reflectors. The bladder was subjected to ballottement by the transducer just before the sonogram was taken. Therefore the particles formed a swirled pattern. The cross section of uterine horn (B) contains a Day-11 conceptus with a specular echo on the upper and lower surfaces.

Shadow Artifacts

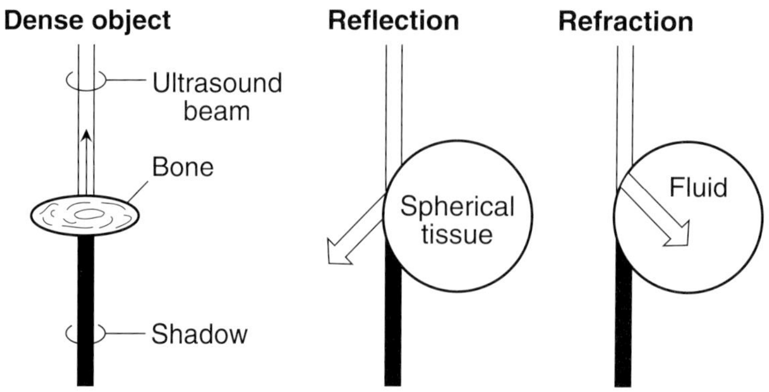

Origin of shadow artifacts. A shadow is caused by blockage or deviation of the sound beams and is comparable to a shadow that occurs behind a light barrier. In the common white-on-black format (pg 59), the area of a sonogram resulting from blocked sound waves appears dark, similar to a shadow resulting from blocked light waves. The shadow shown on the left is caused by reflection of most of the beam back to the transducer, combined with some absorption of the sound by the reflecting structure. Such massive reflections require a marked mismatch in acoustic impedance at the interface between two tissues or entities (e.g., gas and soft tissue; soft tissue and a very dense material, such as bone or a foreign body). The shadow shown in the middle is caused by reflection of the beam from the side of a smooth curved structure (pg 66). Reflection may be the entire reason for beam deviation when the speed of sound is similar in the tissues on both sides of the reflecting surface (e.g., curved side of an ovary or external surface of a cross-section of a uterine horn). However, if there is a mismatch in the speed of sound on each side of the reflecting surface, the portion of the sound pulse that is transmitted through the surface may also undergo refraction (pg 32), as shown on the right. This commonly occurs with fluid-filled structures (e.g., equine yolk sacs, uterine cysts, ovarian follicles). Shadowing, as well as other artifacts, may be more pronounced when the offending object is located in the focal zone; a small object (e.g., 4 mm diameter) may be adequate to block the beam in the narrow focal zone, but not in areas proximal or distal to the focal zone. Blatant shadowing can be caused by fecal material on the face of the probe, and often the debris can be removed with a finger without withdrawing the transducer from the rectum. Defective elements also cause a pronounced vertical band of noninformation that has the appearance of a shadow.

Enhancement Artifacts

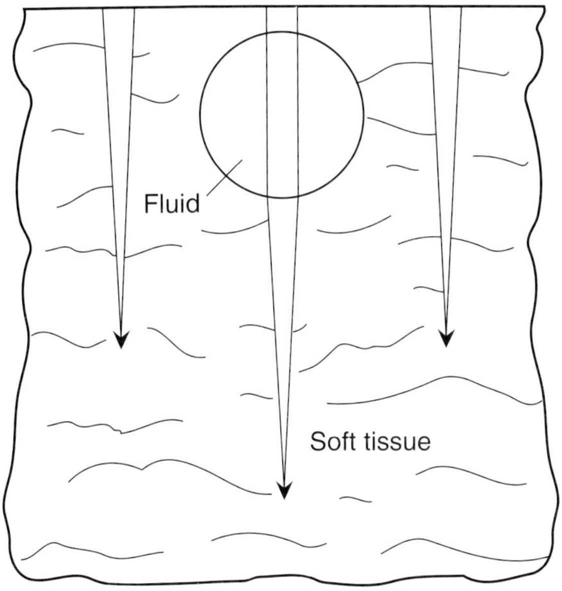

Attenuation of beams and the origin of enhancement artifacts. Enhancement or through-transmission artifacts are common in images of the reproductive tract because of the presence of fluid-filled structures (ovarian follicles, cysts, embryonic vesicles). These artifacts result when the ultrasound beams or pulses pass through a reflector-free structure (i.e., fluid-filled), as shown. The pulse is not depleted (attenuated) by echo production while passing through the fluid; that is, the fluid is anechoic or nonechogenic. Therefore, when the pulse emerges from the far side, the amplitude of the pulse is greater than in the tissues on each side. The relatively greater amplitude or strength of the sound pulses distal to the fluid-filled structure results in a column of relatively brighter echoes beneath the structure.

Enhancement artifacts are often useful because they provide a diagnostic criterion of fluid proximal to the column of enhancement. The sonographer must be careful, however, not to mistake the area of increased echogenicity for a structure (pg 73). Enhancement artifacts tend to obscure the wall of the fluid-filled structure at the point of emergence of the beam. This difficulty is compounded when the wall also produces a specular echo. Such saturation with echo signals in an area of interest can be diminished by adjusting the gain controls to obtain a more reasonable compromise between the saturated area and other areas of interest. The degree of enhancement, as well as shadowing, also can be diminished by using a lower frequency transducer, because ultrasonic attenuation is directly proportional to frequency. In addition, these artifacts will be more pronounced and sharper in the focal zone of the beams.

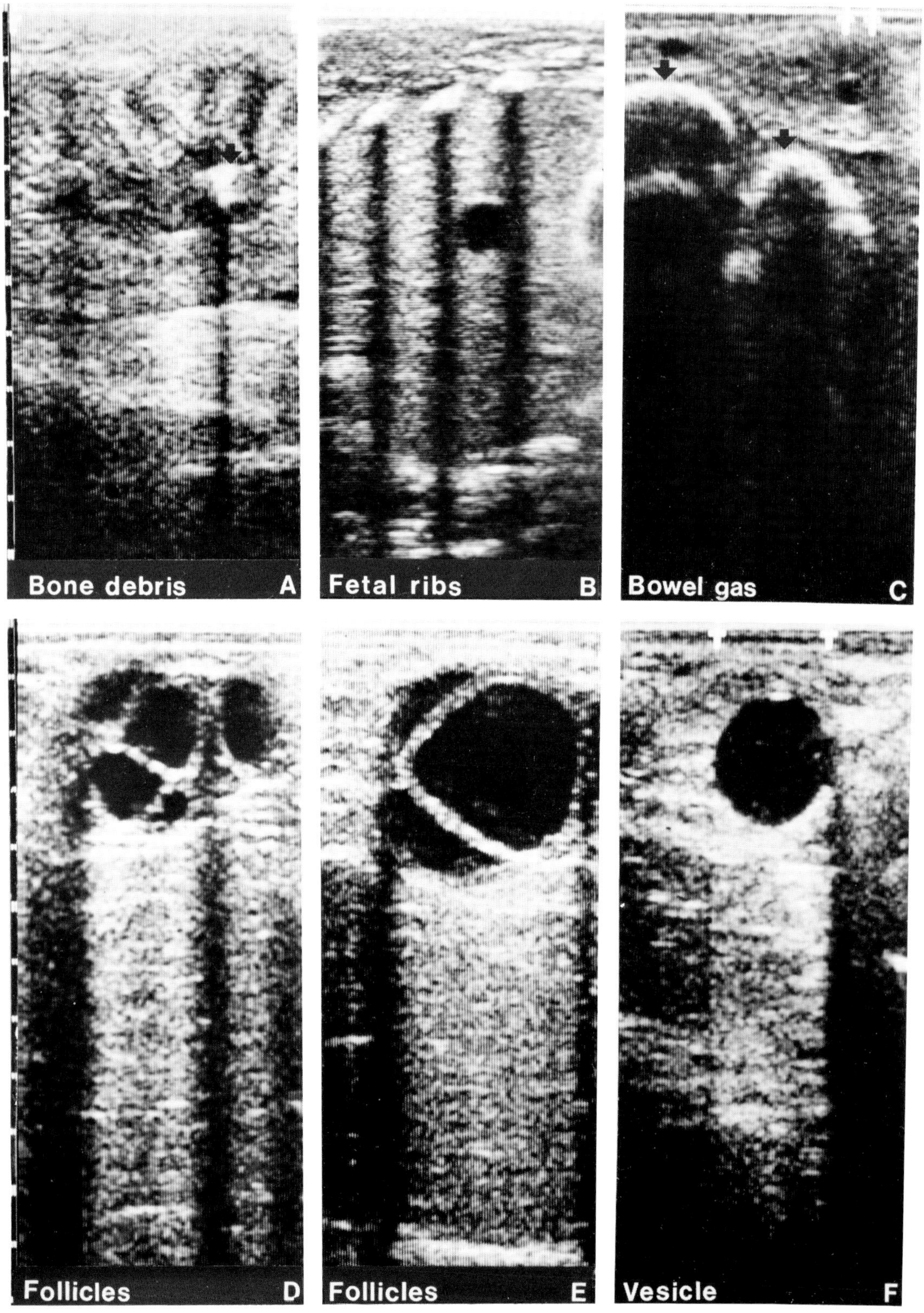
Bone debris A
Fetal ribs B
Bowel gas C
Follicles D
Follicles E
Vesicle F

Examples of shadowing (A-F) and enhancement (D-F) in sonograms from mare reproductive tracts. In sonograms A, B, and C, the shadowing is caused by complete blockage of the ultrasound pulses by very dense or reflective objects. Specifically, the shadowing is due to a fetal bone remnant in the uterus from an abortion (A; arrow), fetal ribs in a normal 120-day conceptus (B), and reflection of the beams from the highly reflective soft tissue and gas interface of two loops of bowel (C; arrows). In D, E, and F, the shadowing is due to reflection and refraction from the sides of follicles and a Day-14 embryonic vesicle. Note the distinct columns of echogenicity (enhancement artifacts) beneath the fluid-filled structures. The enhancement artifacts are accentuated by the columns of shadowing on each side of the column of enhancement, especially in D and E. The enhancement results in greater tissue penetration, as shown by the length and the ultrasonic detail of the echogenic columns. For this reason, the enhancement has been used to project ultrasound beams deeper into a tissue mass by inserting homogenous material (gel, water) or using to advantage a natural fluid-filled structure (e.g., urinary bladder). Shadows and enhancement are major artifacts in images of the female reproductive tract. Shadowing is a problem because the tissue in the involved area is not accessible to imaging unless the sound beam can be adequately redirected. Enhancement is usually not a problem, unless the area of increased echogenicity is mistaken for a structure, as shown below. If enhancement obscures the distal wall of a fluid-filled structure, adjustment of the gain controls will minimize the problem. Shadowing and enhancement are probably as much of a help as a hindrance. Shadows provide information on the density of an offending object and may delineate the lateral boundaries of a round, solid structure. Either artifact may serve to draw the operator's attention to a fluid-filled or other homogeneous structure.

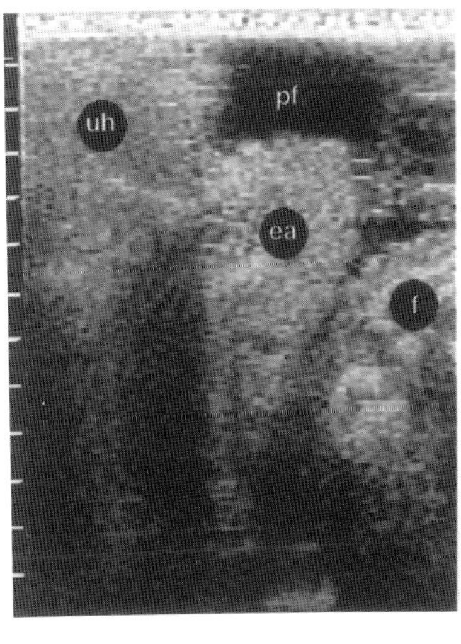

Misleading enhancement. ea=enhancement artifact. f=fetus. pf=placental fluid. uh=uterine horn. Initially the enhancement of the uterine tissue in the uterine intercornual area during pregnancy was mistaken for an area of denser tissue and therefore was identified as the internal intercornual ligament. This error was corrected by considering the principals of artifactual responses, especially the effect of placental fluid above the hyperechogenic area.

Reverberation Artifacts

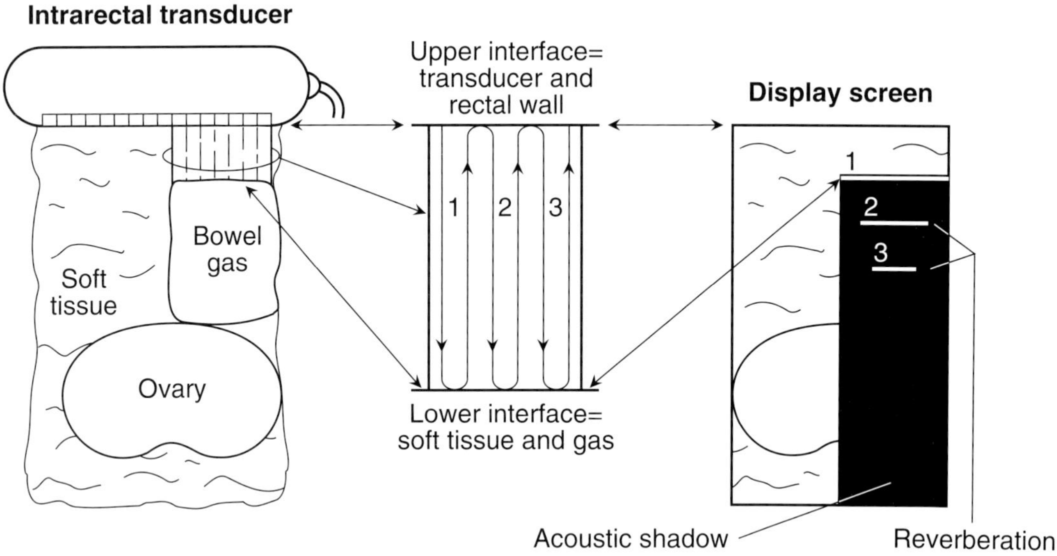

Origin of reverberation artifacts. Reverberation is a process wherein an echo bounces between two strong interfaces until the ultrasound pulses are exhausted by attenuation. The illustration shows the origin of reverberation artifacts on the display screen as a result of the sound waves bouncing between a soft tissue-gas interface and the interface consisting of the transducer and rectal wall. The pulse is shown making three round trips between interfaces. Round trip number l results in a legitimate echo on the display screen (echo l). The second and third trips, however, result in false or reverberation marks on the screen. At the completion of the first round trip, the echo strikes the transducer crystals and produces a small voltage, which in turn results in an echo at the appropriate pixel on the screen. However, much of the sound energy is reflected back into the tissue, because the transducer-rectal wall interface represents a profound acoustic impedance mismatch and therefore a very effective ultrasonic reflector. On the second return trip, the pulse again strikes the crystals, resulting in another echo on the screen (echo 2). This time, however, the scan converter assigns an address that is twice as far from the top of the screen (representing the transducer face) as for the legitimate echo; the second trip resulted in a doubling of the interval from the time the pulse originally left the transducer (trip l) until the echo struck the transducer after trip 2. In addition, the amplitude of the second echo is weaker because of additional attenuation. Therefore the resulting echo on the screen is not as distinct as the first. If there is sufficient amplitude remaining after the second trip, this process may continue producing additional echo signals that are equidistant from one another but progressively weaker. Because of the resulting decreasing strength of the reverberations, these are sometimes called comet-tail artifacts *(25)*. Three distinguishing features help identify reverberation artifacts: 1) they are equidistant, 2) they gradually diminish in intensity, and 3) they are oriented parallel to the reflective interface.

If a very reflective interface is involved (soft tissue/gas), none of the pulse is transmitted through the interface. Therefore, an acoustic shadow results and the reverberation echoes on the screen are placed in the shadow. If part of the pulse is transmitted, as in a soft tissue/liquid interface, the resulting reverberations are placed in the nonechogenic image of the fluid. The more reflective the interface, the greater the likelihood of reverberations. In addition, when the reflective interface is close to the transducer, attenuation is minimal, and the number and intensity of reverberations are increased. Reverberation artifacts are more likely to be seen when they are contrasted with an acoustic shadow or nonechogenic fluid. However, they may be present also in the more echogenic portions of the image and may not be noticed because they are masked.

Reverberation artifacts are very common in the pelvic area because of pockets of bowel gas. In addition, the many fluid-filled structures in the reproductive tract increase the potential for legible reverberations. Reverberation echoes within fluid-filled structures would be troublesome because they could be mistaken for echoes representing internal structure. Sometimes the distance from transducer to the surface of a fluid-filled structure is too great and the reflective properties of the structure are not adequate to produce visible reverberation echoes. Apparently, reverberation artifacts can appear on an image even though the source of the reverberations (bowel gas, pelvic bone) is beneath the displayed depth of the image. The echoes from such structures may reach the transducer after another pulse has been emitted. In this event, the reverberation marks would be superimposed on the image resulting from the subsequent beams, and the origin of the reverberations would not be apparent. Some of the unexplained, bright echoes on images of this body area may be from this source.

Internal reverberations also can occur due to rebounding between two interfaces within the animal's tissue (e.g., within fluid-filled structures). The resulting artifacts are difficult to distinguish from real echoes.

Since continuing reverberation depends on adequate signal amplitude, the number and brightness of reverberation artifacts increase as the gain is increased. Appropriate adjustment of the gain controls may help diminish the reverberation problem. In addition to proper gain control adjustments, reverberations sometimes can be minimized by manually reorienting the organs of interest (ovaries, uterus) in relation to the offending loops of bowel. Multiple reverberations with distinct shadowing often are caused by fecal fluid between the transducer and the rectal wall. This problem usually can be corrected by reorienting the transducer.

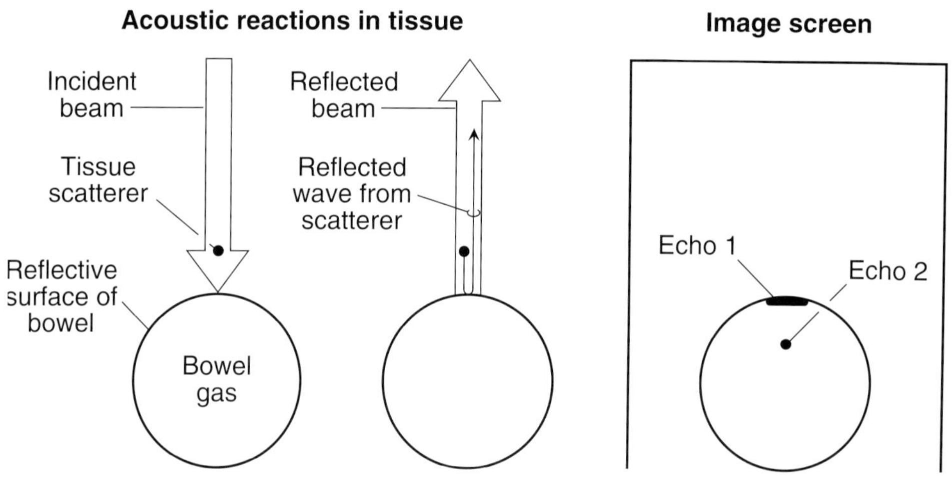

Origin of artifactual scattered echoes in a reverberation path. Scattered echo signals often appear beyond highly reflective surfaces between a tissue reflector and the first reverberation echo or between successive reverberation echoes. The origin of the artifactual patterns *(179)* is depicted. When the incident beam traverses the soft tissue, scatters are encountered, which produce nonspecular echoes as described elsewhere (pg 68). When the incident beam strikes the highly reflective surface, a large fraction of its energy is reflected. The reflected beam also encounters the scatterers when returning toward the transducer. Some of the resulting waves from the scatterers also reflect off the highly reflective surface, as shown. These latter echoes (echo 2) trail the main echo (echo 1) back to the transducer. The scanner, therefore, places the origin of the diffuse echoes beyond the reflecting surface. Examples of artifactual echoes in reverberation paths are shown in the following ultrasonograms.

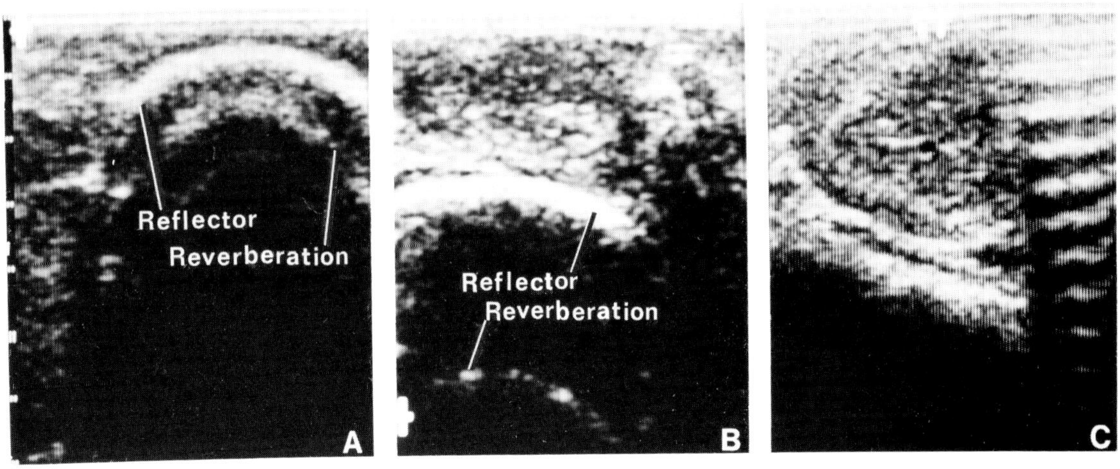

Examples of reverberation echoes. In sonograms A and B, the reverberation echo originates from a reflection off the surface of a gas-filled loop of bowel. Note for both A and B that the distance from transducer face (top of image) to the reflector is equal to the distance from reflector to the reverberation echo and that the reverberations fall within the shadow cast by the reflecting surface. In C, the comet-tail reverberations (right side of image) probably resulted from a film of fecal fluid between the transducer face and the rectal wall. Note that the reverberation echoes are equidistant and progressively weaker. The reverberation echoes in A and B are curved because the highly reflective surface of the air-filled bowel is curved. In contrast, the reverberation echoes in C are straight, because the contact areas between the transducer face, intervening material, and rectal wall are straight. Artifactual echoes due to scatters, as described above, are prominent beneath the reflector (A, B).

Beam-width Artifacts

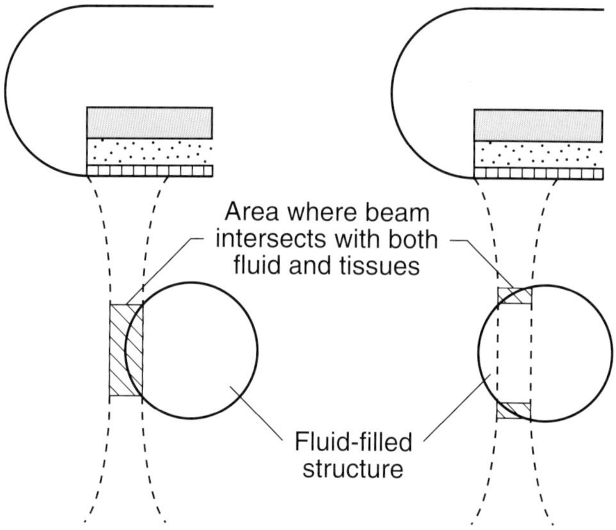

Origin of beam-width artifacts. The periphery of large, fluid-filled structures or the entire fluid volume of a small structure often casts a foggy appearance due to partial fill-in of the nonechogenic fluid with echogenic artifactual spots. As a result, the expected sharp, distinct outline is not obtained. The lack of detail is especially noticeable on the lateral walls (with respect to the image) of the fluid-filled structures. As shown above, this is a problem of lateral resolution resulting from portions of the beam sampling both wall and fluid at a given depth *(178)*. When two echoes reach the transducer at the same time, they are treated as one echo and result in one signal. Because the beam fans out beyond the focal zone, beam-width artifacts sometimes appear at the bottom of large structures (e.g., preovulatory equine follicle). Such artifacts may assume a meniscus-like shape, resulting from a change in the solid:fluid ratio as the beams move along the linear array of elements *(174)*. Beam-width artifacts can be generated not only in the plane of the scan or image (width of field of view), but also in the opposite plane corresponding to the thickness of the ultrasonic slice of tissue *(178)*. Beam-width artifacts can mimic solid projections *(146)* or disorganization of the wall. If beam-width artifacts are misinterpreted as an indication of partial collapse or disorganization of the wall, an erroneous conclusion of impending ovulation, follicular atresia, or embryonic death may be made. The origin of echogenic spots within a fluid-filled structure sometimes can be determined by ballottement of the structure with the transducer; true reflectors may respond by floating. Since the artifact is a function of beam width, the artifactual fill-in can be reduced by using a transducer that has a narrower beam at the depth of greatest interest.

As noted above, beam width also contributes to shadowing (pg 70) and enhancement artifacts (pg 71). In the focal zone, the beam is narrow and the intensity of the sound pulses is great. Solid structures (bone) and fluid-filled structures that interact with the beam in the focal zone produce more intense artifacts. In addition, the small offending structures are more likely to involve the entire width of the beam in the focal zone. Occasionally, a band-like artifactual area of increased echogenicity is observed in the focal zone when scanning large solid structures.

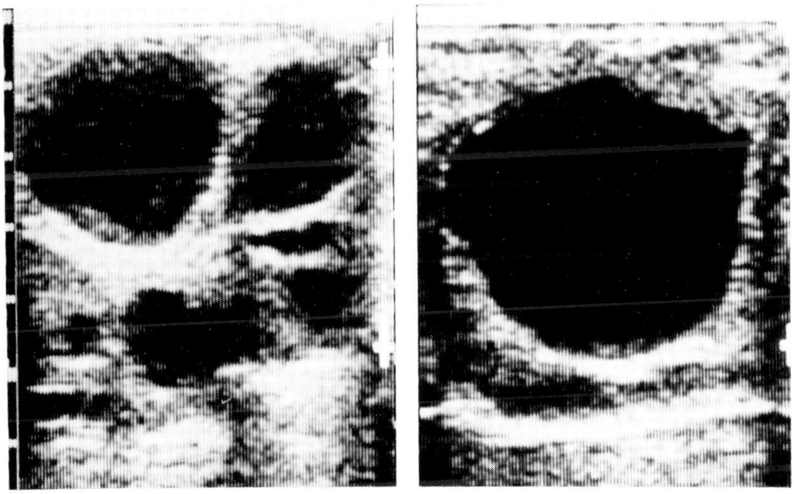

Examples of apparent beam-width artifacts. Note the echoes scattered near the periphery of the fluid-filled equine follicles (left) and near the bottom of an embryonic vesicle (right). Perhaps the echogenic spots on the bottom of the embryonic vesicle are due to a curvature of the vesicle in the plane associated with the thickness of the ultrasonic slice; the curvature in the width plane does not seem to adequately account for a beam-width artifact.

Other Artifacts

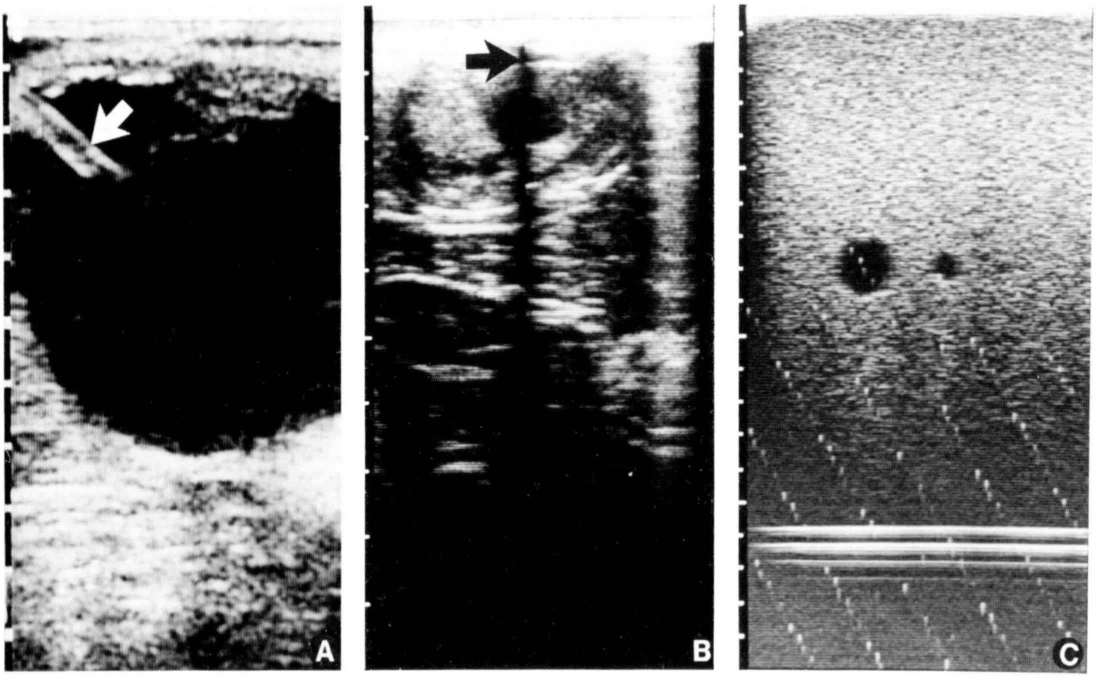

Examples of artifacts due to faulty equipment or outside interference. Ultrasound scanners are highly complex, and the images are subject to aberrations due to engineering flaws or shortcuts, malfunctioning, and outside electrical interference.

(A) The diagonal bright column (arrow) was due to the engineering design of the transducer. Sometimes there are trade-offs in design, so that maximal achievement of one goal is done at the expense of another. Apparently, some scanner models are engineered to provide a sensitive response to minute tissue differences and therefore are subject to more artifacts. Other models, for example, may be programmed to block out anechoic areas in an exaggerated manner to give esthetically pleasing images of fluid areas, but at the expense of subtle, detailed information concerning the fluid area.

(B) The dark vertical line was due to improper contact between the connection of the transducer's coaxial cable and the receptacle in the console. It was corrected by proper seating. A similar black line can be caused by malfunctioning elements at the origin of the line.

(C) The noise (diagonal, bright lines) was due to electrical interference from attempting to run another scanner on the same electric circuit. Refrigerators and dairy milking units are a common source of such interference. Sonogram C was made by imaging an ultrasonic tissue phantom. The bright horizontal lines near the bottom of the image represent the phantom design and are not artifacts. Large shadows or fluid-filled structures (cysts, embryonic vesicles) serve as good test areas for the presence of extraneous signals. If the shadow or fluid contains echogenic areas that do not appear to be caused by reverberations or beam-width artifacts, electric noise or engineering artifacts may be superimposed on the picture. Such noise may be present, but not noticeable, in the more echogenic portions of the image.

Consult literature sources *(e.g., 25, 48, 106, 176)* for descriptions and discussions of other artifacts. For example, multipath artifacts can occur when an ultrasound beam undergoes multiple reflections; false echoes can be placed on the screen for echoes that are able to return to the transducer. An artifact due to velocity differences in the tissues is another example; when the velocity of the medium between two imaged interfaces is different from the standardized velocity (1540 m/s), the spacing between the interfaces on the screen will be in error. Spurious echo signals produced by multiple reflections and complexities are not readily explained. Artifacts may result not only from the nature of beam propagation and interaction with the tissue and electronic ramifications but also from scan-converter and display considerations *(106)*. Considering the myriad of extraneous phenomena that can activate the crystals of the transducer or the pixels of the TV screen, the ultrasonographer should not expect to account for every signal on the screen. Perhaps the real wonder is that ultrasonic scanners present so much useful information, despite the apparent chaos as the pulses pass and bounce through the tissues.

Nonechogenicity

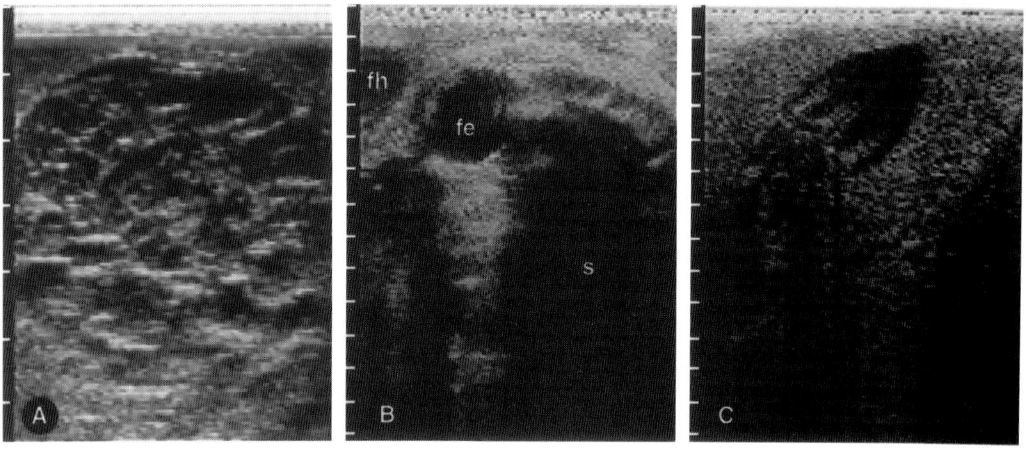

Examples of anechoic structures.

(A) Blood clot in an unovulated equine follicle. The black areas (anechoic) interspersed among the web-like echogenic bands represent areas of firm clotted material.

(B) Anechoic areas from the tip of a fetal hoof (fh) and fetal eye (fe) with shadowing (s) beneath the fetal head. The hoof is from a rear limb encased in the uterine horn and is separated from the fetal head by walls of the tip of the uterine horn and the uterine body *(64)*.

(C) Fetal equine hoof encased in a uterine horn as in image B. The anechoic area is from solid, homogeneous material.

In the white-on-black format, when a structure reflects all the sound waves, the areas distal to the structure will not receive waves, and therefore are black (shadowing; pg 70), as shown in sonogram B. Similarly, structures devoid of reflectors will appear black on a properly adjusted scanner screen. It is often thought that anechoic structures are necessarily fluid filled. This is erroneous. Nonechogenicity occurs in solids as well as fluids. The only requirement for nonechogenicity is uniformity of fluid or tissue makeup so that reflecting interfaces are absent or inconsequential. There are many anechoic fluid-filled structures in the female reproductive tract (e.g., pg 10). A few nonfluid structures of the reproductive tract, however, are anechoic, as shown above. The fetal hoof (C) is of special interest because, when originally observed, the anechoic area was assumed to represent placental fluid surrounding the fetal limbs. Study of a removed fetus, however, clarified that the black anechoic area was hoof and the uterine horn encasing the limbs did not contain detectable placental fluid *(64)*.

Part Two

EQUIPMENT

Chapter 6

SCANNERS

The encouragement in Chapter 5 to develop and hone image-interpreting abilities assumes the availability of images worth trying to interpret. This chapter provides information on the selection, operation, and care of scanners with a view toward attaining high-quality images. Examples are shown of linear-array transducers, and attention is given to transducer care and maintenance. Transducer frequency is discussed with the aid of sonograms from scans of ultrasonic phantoms. The console and its manual adjustments are considered with emphasis on the contrast, brightness, and gain controls. A section is included on the use of phantoms for assessing and monitoring scanner and transducer quality. The capabilities of scanners used in human medicine are discussed briefly as a representation of the current status of the technology when cost is not the major limitation.

Some veterinary ultrasound scanners are still being sold that are high in price, but low in quality. A potential buyer is faced with selecting a make and model suitable to specific needs. This chapter includes a section on considerations for instrument selection. Photographic examples of available transducers and scanners are included. Use of images prepared from a given make and model or photographs or other references to specific models should not be taken as a recommendation for purchase. Our laboratory has used instruments that were loaned to us or provided at a reduced cost for research. The photographs of instruments in this chapter were prepared by us, except as noted, using scanners available when the photographs were taken.

The Transducer

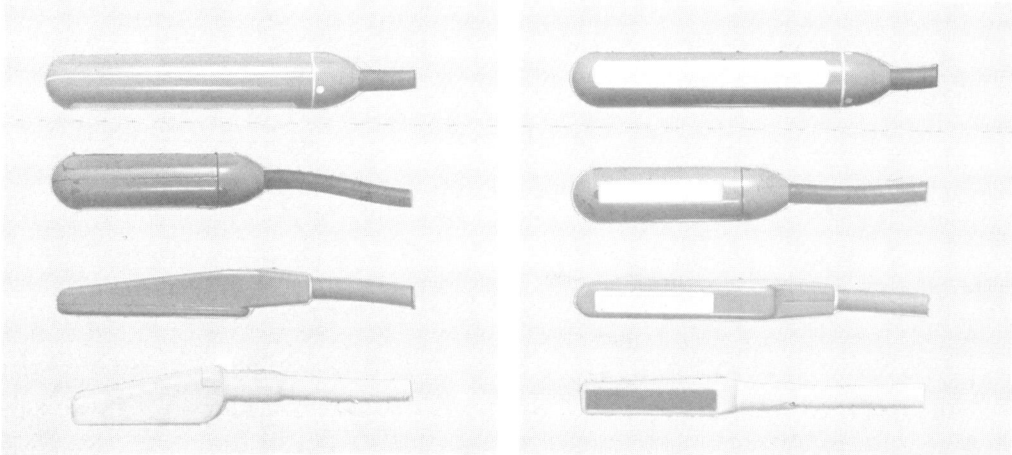

Examples of linear-array transducers. Side (left) and face (right) views are shown (25% of actual size). The linear array of crystals is located beneath the rectangular areas on the face views.

Intrarectal transducers must be designed for ease of insertion and manipulation and for minimization of trauma. However, the instrument should have adequate bulk and grip for easy manipulation and to prevent hand cramping during prolonged use. One should be able to digitally identify the active surface. Transducers should be waterproof and resistant to corrosion. Transducers that require insertion into a plastic cover before intrarectal use are undesirable. Waterproofing and electric insulation are important to prevent electric shocks to the animal or operator and damage to the delicate interior of the transducer. In this regard, users should consider the chance of damage to the scanner, operator, and animal during lightning storms. Although transducers are complex and refined instruments, they also must be durable for animal use.

The coaxial cable connects the transducer to the console. The cable must attach to the end of the probe for intrarectal use, as shown, but for transcutaneous applications the cable can attach opposite to the face, as shown elsewhere (pg 104, pg 109). The cable contains many fine electric wires because of the necessity for independent connections to each crystal. The junction of the cable and transducer must be well-insulated and sealed. The cable should be flexible for intrarectal use and must not be bulky; a thick cable will interfere with intrarectal manipulations and will cause discomfort to the forearm resulting from the action of the anal sphincter. On most scanners, the cables are too long and drag on the floor when the operator works with the animal close to the scanner (pg 132). The intrarectal transducer should be withdrawn from the rectum by the gripping hand and not by pulling on the cable.

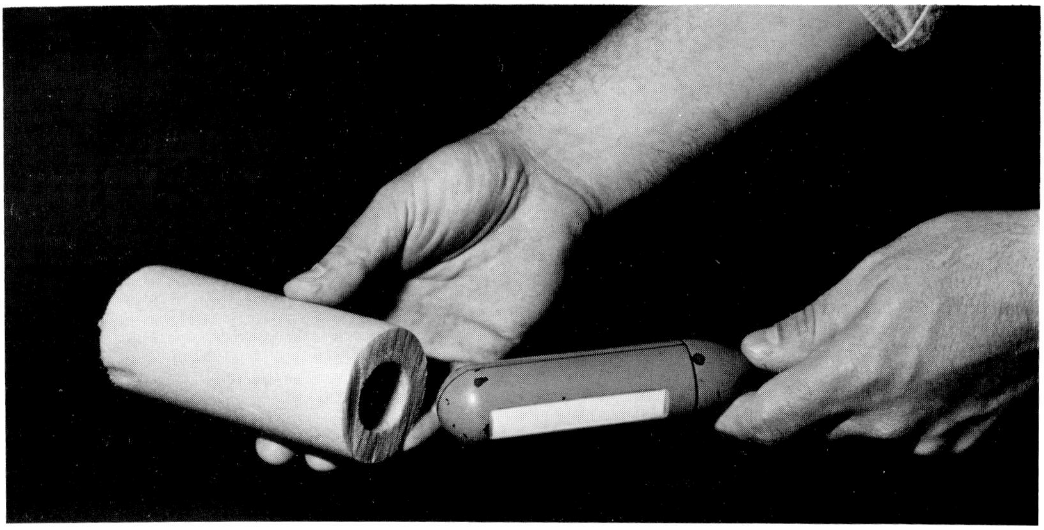

Insertion of a transducer into a protective sleeve. Transducers are precision instruments and expensive ($3,000 to $8,000) and must be handled with care. Dropping the instrument or marring the covering over the elements can cause a malfunction, and a cracked transducer could cause an electric shock *(179)*. The ceramic crystals are brittle, and there are many connecting points of fine wire within the transducer. A defective element or connector may result in a vertical, spurious line through the image corresponding to the defective area (pg 80). When the transducer is not being held, provision is needed to hang or secure it, so that it does not drop accidentally onto a hard surface. An effective method is shown for protecting the transducer when not in use. A length of the foam cylinders that are used to insulate water pipes is obtained from a hardware or plumber's store. If the optimum diameter is used, the transducer is easily inserted, yet the cover will stay firmly in place and provide a thick, protective cushion. The transducer is washed and dried before insertion into the protective transport cylinder. Coupling gel will dry onto the transducer and should be removed with a soft towel. Occasionally, one may wish to examine a portion of the reproductive tract during surgery (pg 138). For such use, the transducer should be cold-sterilized (e.g., with ethylene oxide) according to the recommendations of the manufacturer. A preferred method is to insert the probe into a sterile plastic sleeve along with coupling gel. Autoclaving or heating to temperatures of 100° C may not affect the properties of the crystals but could have a drastic effect on the bonding cements *(106)*.

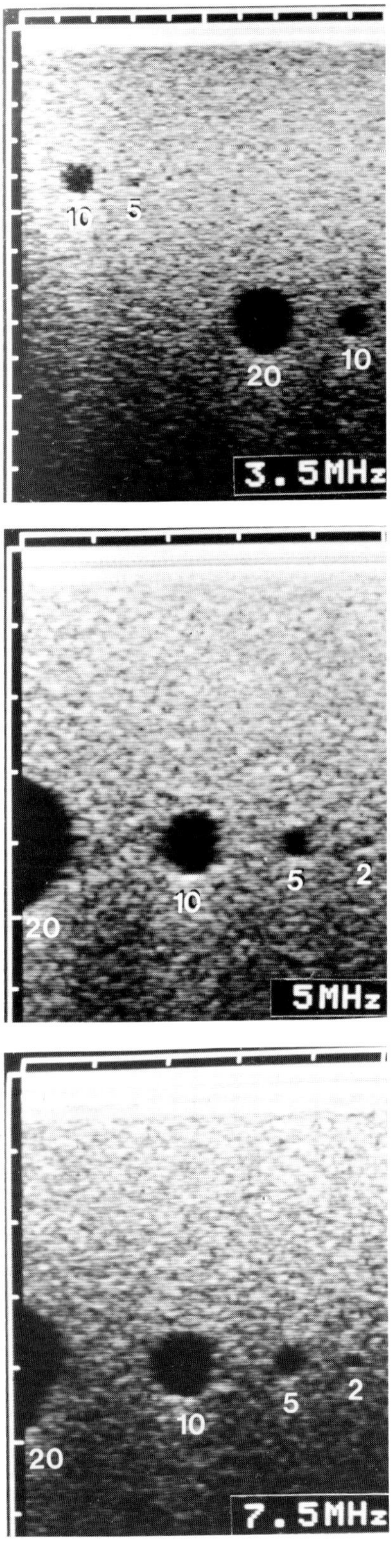

Images for various transducer frequencies. The sonograms compare the resolutions and penetrations of 3.5, 5.0, and 7.5 MHz transducers. The medium is an ultrasonic phantom, and the nonechogenic objects are cross-sections of fluid-filled cylinders with the indicated diameters. The scale is in centimeters. The centers of the cross-sectional views are at depths of 4 cm and 8 cm. The 3.5 MHz transducer barely defines the 5 mm object and does not detect the 2 mm object. The greater resolution of the 5.0 MHz transducer is demonstrated by the clearly defined 5 mm object and the barely defined 2 mm object. The 7.5 MHz transducer provides additional resolution, as indicated by the improved definition of the 2 mm object. However, the penetration of the 3.5 MHz transducer is much greater than that of the other transducers. The 20 mm object at 8 cm was clearly visible with the 3.5 MHz transducer but barely visible with the others (not shown). The 10 mm object is more distinct at 8 cm than at 4 cm with the 3.5 MHz transducer. The hazy appearance at 4 cm is attributable to beam-width artifacts (pg 78) because the focal zone is beyond the object. These comparisons demonstrate that the focal depths of the 5.0 MHz and 3.5 MHz transducers were close to 4 cm and 8 cm, respectively. Engineering modifications have been made in some models so that the field of view of the 7.5 MHz transducer is comparable to that of the 5.0 MHz transducer, despite the increased frequency and improved resolving power.

Item	3.5 MHz transducer	5.0 MHz transducer
Minimum follicle diameter	6-8 mm	2-3 mm
Detectability of corpus luteum	For 5-6 days	Day 0 to regression
Earliest detection of conceptus	Day 11 (6-7 mm)	Day 9 or 10 (3-4 mm)

Effect of frequency on detectability. The difference in resolving power between a 3.5 MHz and 5.0 MHz transducer can be appreciated in the detectability of structures in the reproductive tract.

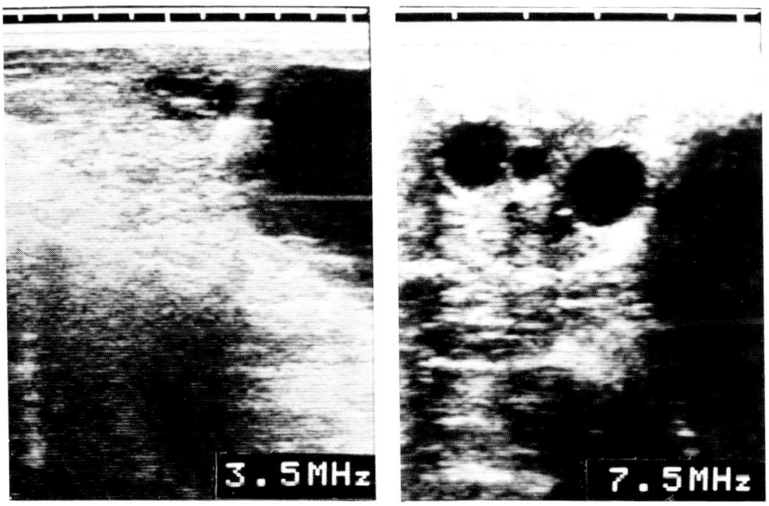

Ultrasonograms of an equine ovary taken with 3.5 and 7.5 MHz transducers. The resolving capabilities of the 7.5 MHz transducer were much greater than those of the 3.5 MHz transducer. The focal point of the 3.5 MHz transducer greatly exceeds the 2 cm distance from transducer to center of ovary. This comparison further illustrates the advantage of the higher frequency transducers, noted on the previous page. The distance from the transducer face during transrectal imaging to the center of the ovary or the lumen of a nongravid uterus is only a few centimeters. Therefore, a higher frequency transducer (e.g., 5.0 MHz) with a focal point of 3 or 4 cm is well suited for intrarectal examination of the reproductive tract in nonpregnant or early pregnant large animals. The lower frequency transducers (e.g., 3.5 MHz) are more suited for examining the uterus during late pregnancy or soon after parturition.

The Console

Aloka
210

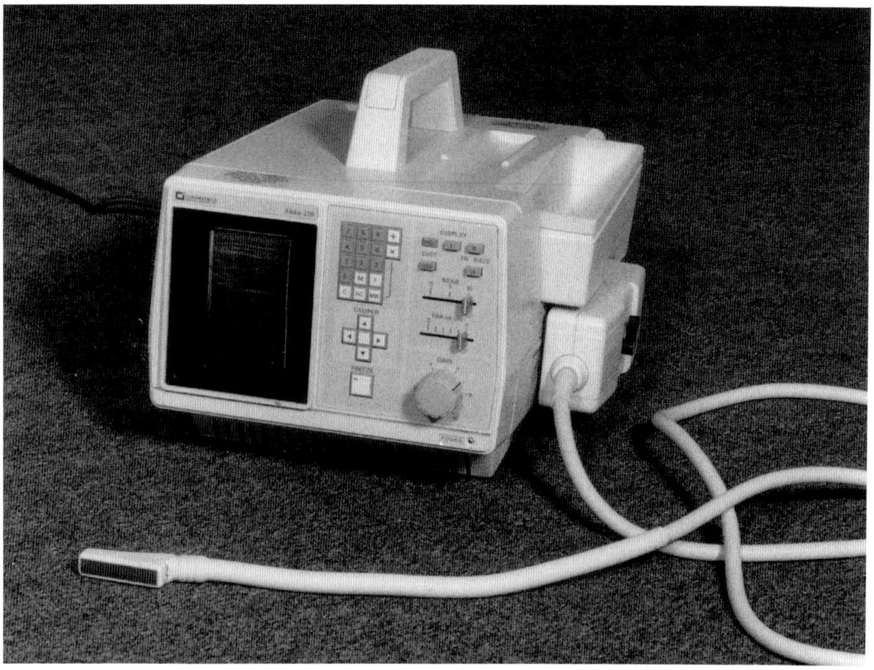

Aloka
500

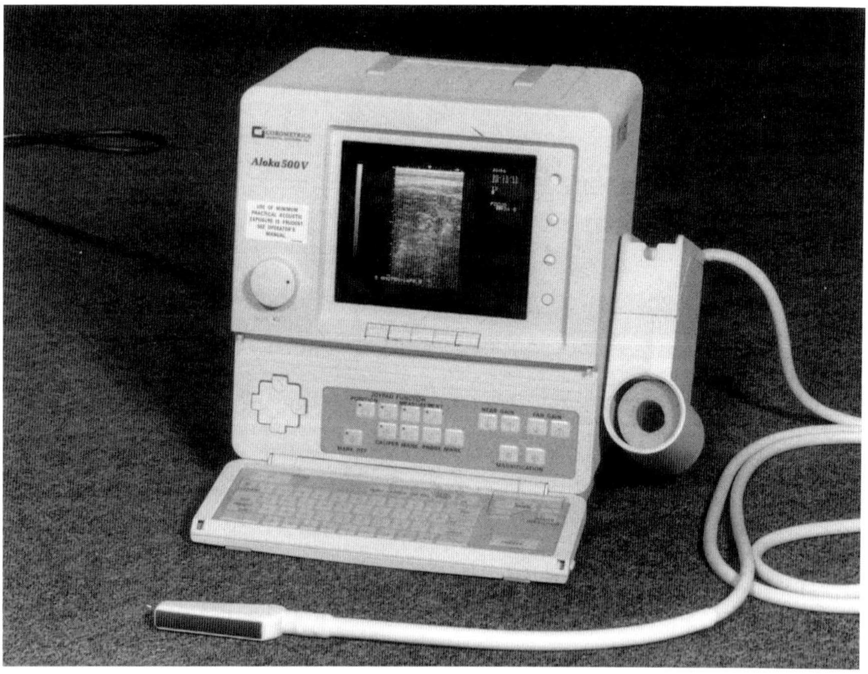

Examples of ultrasound scanners (pgs 90 to 93). Previous models (upper) and latest models (lower) are shown for Aloka (pg 90), Pie Medical (pg 91), and Tokyo Keiki (pg 92) and the latest model from Dynamic Imaging (pg 93; source information: pg 191). For sonography in animals, portability is important because the scanner may be moved from farm to farm or from animal to animal on a given farm.

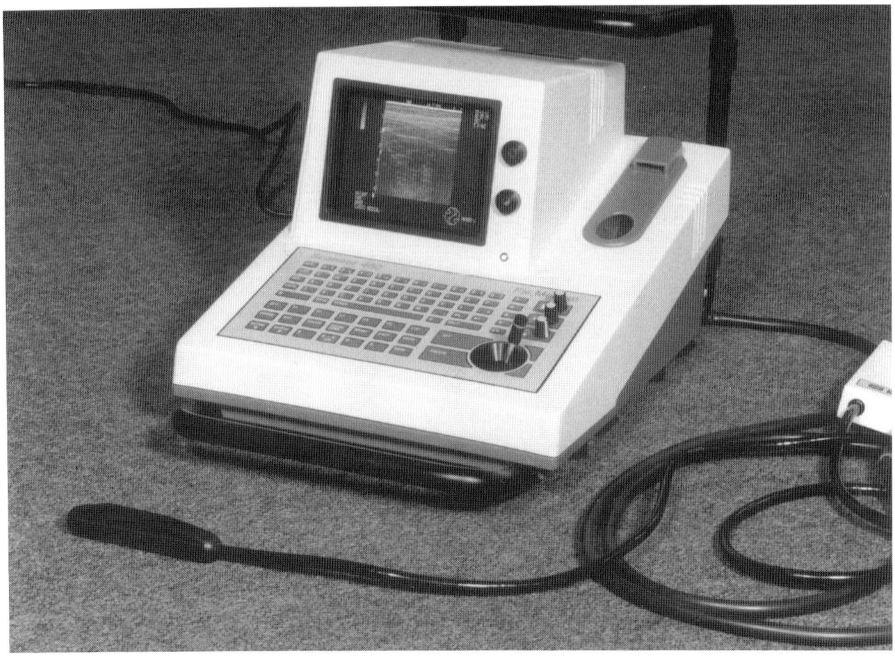

Pie Medical 480

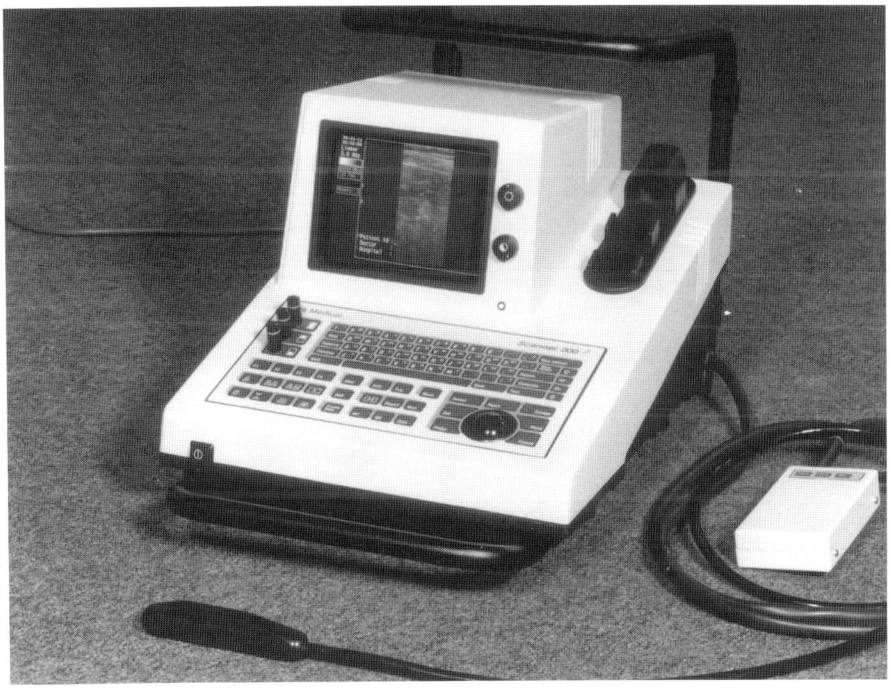

Pie Medical 200

Therefore scanners are equipped with a handle and other provisions for transport. Examples of weights of models are 10 kg (22 lbs, Aloka 500) and 7 kg (15 lbs, Ultrascan II). Despite the complexity of the console, it should be durable and require minimal servicing. A clear plastic film can be fastened over the face to prevent dirt or manure from entering and caking around the buttons.

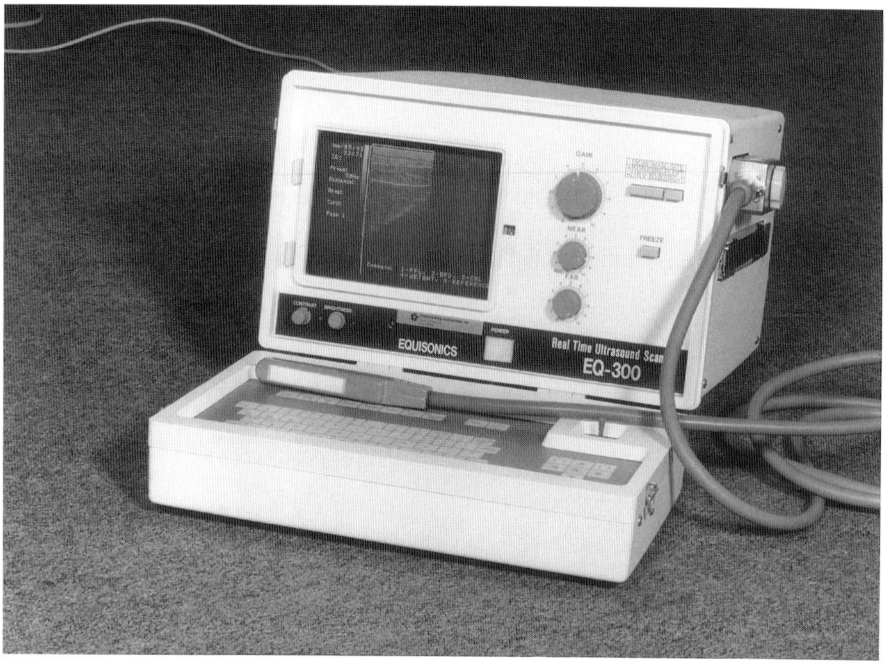

Tokyo Keiki 300

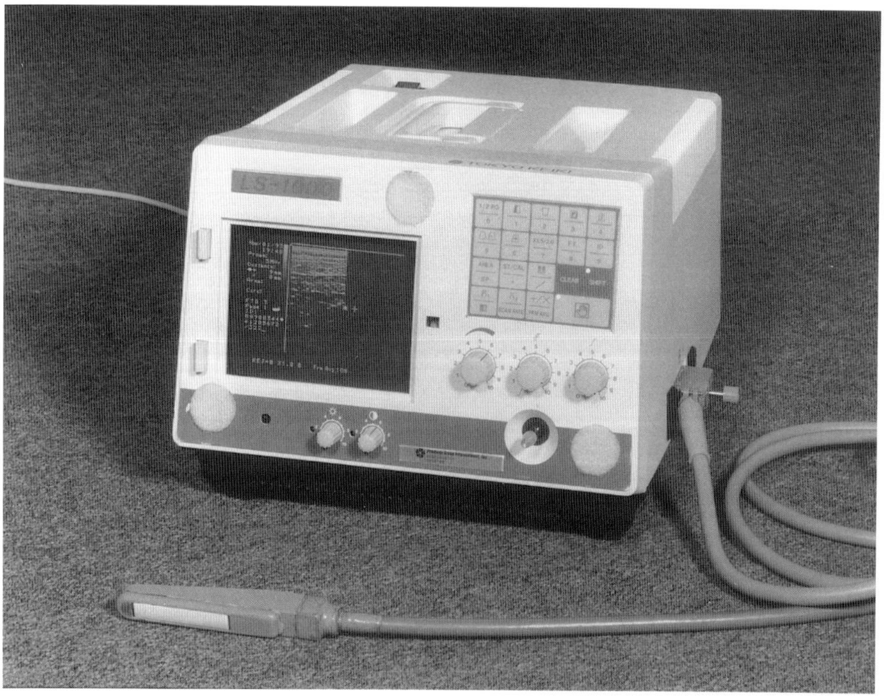

Tokyo Keiki 1000

Most models have near, far, and overall gain controls, a magnification or zoom feature, a freeze button, brightness and contrast controls, and electronic calipers. The brightness and contrast controls are usually knobs or press buttons on the front panel or may be on the side or rear of the console and adjusted with a

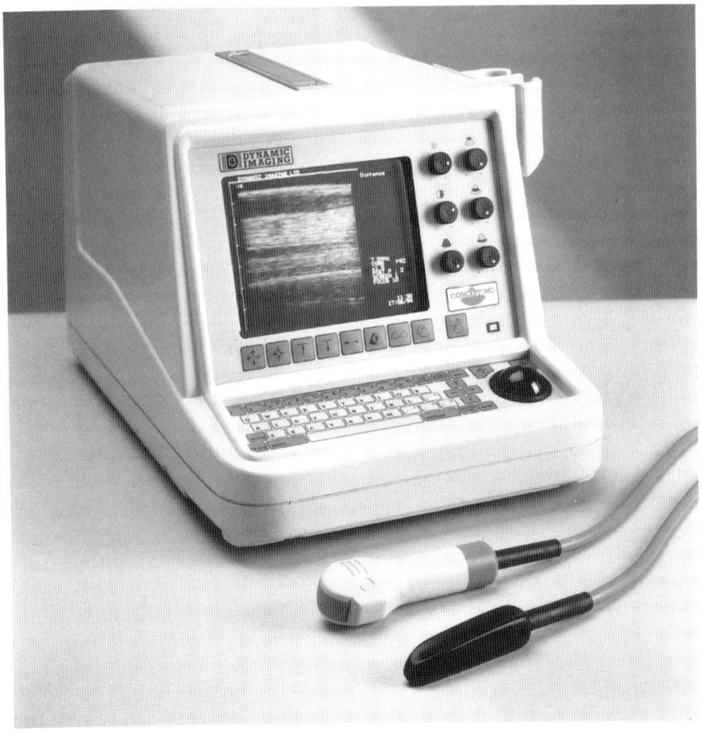

Dynamic Imaging

Photograph courtesy of Products Group International, Inc.

screwdriver or special tool. On some models, the integral electronic calipers for measuring linear distances and areas are controlled by omnidirectional press switches. Toggle and trackerball controls also are used and are preferable because they are faster and more maneuverable. The keyboard is for making annotations on the image to permanently identify videotapes and photographs (e.g., animal and farm identity, date, operator, day of pregnancy).

Various annotation schemes and pull-down menus or windows are provided with different makes of scanners. A simplified and less expensive system is probably adequate for most purposes. Systems are becoming available that allow operators to program their own data (e.g., diameter of fetal eye for estimating days of pregnancy) into the console. The usefulness and accuracy of preprogrammed and self-programmed data (e.g., estimations of fetal age) are limited by biological variation and operator variation.

The console of an ultrasound scanner should not be opened by an inexperienced technician. There is risk of electric shock even after the power cord is disconnected. The scanner switch should be in the off position whenever the power outlet is to be connected or disconnected, apparently to avoid damage resulting from the sudden electric surge. An adapter can be added to the electric plug to minimize potential harmful effects of spurious electric surges.

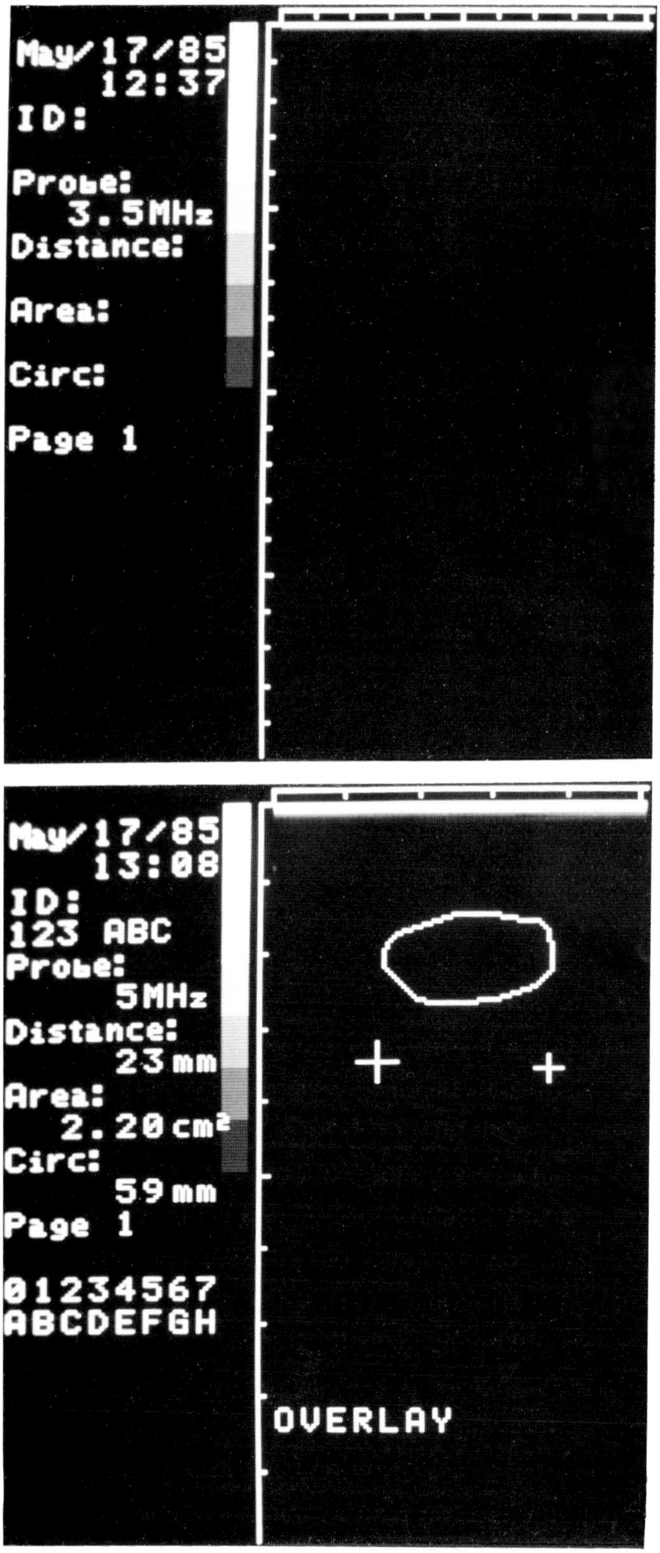

Viewing screen showing the shade bar, annotations, and centimeter scale for a 3.5 MHz and a 5.0 MHz transducer. The screen is devoid of echoes. The brightness control affects the amount of light associated with echoes on the screen. This control may be increased until light just begins to appear on the screen. Contrast is adjusted until all segments of the gray-scale shade bar are clear or until the darkest bar just begins to come into view. Shade bars are provided on the screen for this purpose; a segmental gray-scale with a discrete marker for each shade seems more useful than gradual scales. Proper adjustment of the contrast assures that the operator is using the maximum range of the gray scale. As noted above, contrast and brightness are preset or adjusted with a tool on some older scanners.

The 3.5 MHz screen shows the labeling categories and the automatic recording of date and time. Examples of annotations made by keyboard entries are shown on the 5.0 MHz screen. The electronic caliper markers were placed on the screen by the operator and the distance between them (23 mm) was recorded automatically. The accuracy of electronic calipers involves a fraction of a millimeter *(179)*, but in practice considerable error may be introduced by uncertainty or inconsistency in placement.

Cross-sectional areas can be measured with an error of approximately 5% *(179)*, but error is increased by difficulties in precise steering of the calipers. Volume may be estimated by measuring a number of cross-sectional areas and applying an appropriate mathematical formula. Height of fluid-filled structures is more accurately determined than width; the upper and lower specular echoes serve as distinct markers when height is measured, whereas the side of the structure may be obscured by artifacts (pg 73). An imaginary structure was outlined in the above illustration and the area is given.

Image Inversion

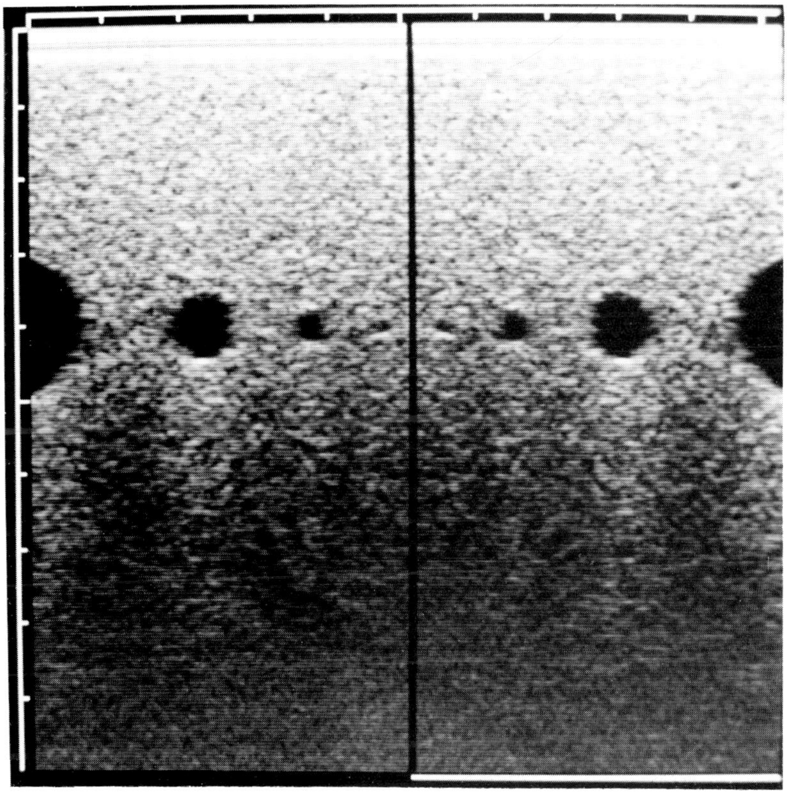

An original and an inverted image. Some scanners are equipped with an inversion control, so that the images can be oriented with the cranial aspect of the tissues either to the left or right of the viewing screen. This capability allows the ultrasonographer to more readily associate the image with the orientation of the tissues being viewed (pg 131). It is convenient to have the caudal aspect of the tissues appear on the right of the screen when the scanner is placed obliquely on the right of the operator and to the left of the screen when the scanner is on the left. The inversion setting can easily be tested by sliding a finger over the face of the transducer.

Gain Controls

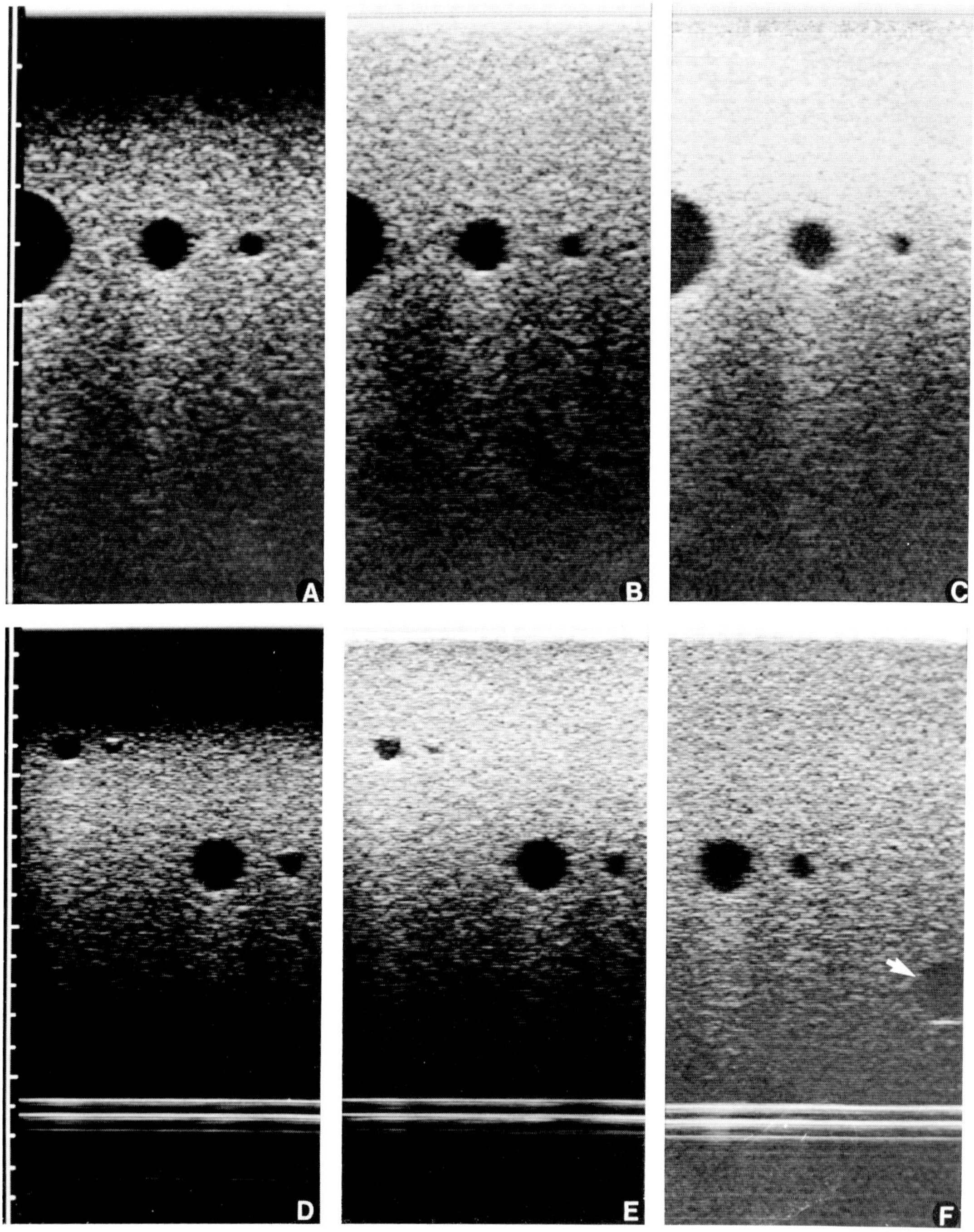

Examples of various gain settings (facing page). Proper adjustment of the gain controls is crucial to building a balanced, pleasing image. The gain adjustments equalize the signal amplitude at various depths (pg 54). When the amplifier gain is too high, the echoes are too strong and the display is overloaded. Conversely, if the gain is too low, the echoes are inadequate. The sonograms were taken with a 5.0 MHz (A,B,C) or 3.5 MHz (D,E,F) transducer and a scanner that had controls for overall, near, and far gain. A,D) Overall gain adjusted to an optimum level, but near gain is too low; objects in the first 2 cm (A) or 4 cm (D) from the transducer would not be detected or would just begin to come into view. B,E) Same as A and D, but near gain now is adjusted. C) Overall gain too high; note that the cross-sectional views of the cylinders have lost their normal anechoic (black) appearance. This same problem would occur if the brightness control were set too high. F) Far gain has been increased so that the 20 mm object at 12 cm is just beginning to come into view (arrow).

Usually, the gain controls can be adjusted at the beginning of the examination of a number of animals with no adjustment thereafter except for occasional fine-tuning. All controls (brightness, contrast, gain) must be considered together. The adjustment of the brightness control of the screen, for example, directly influences the optimal setting for the gain controls of the console. A systematic adjustment procedure can be used, followed by fine-tuning during examinations. One systematic approach is as follows:

1. Turn all controls down.

2. Adjust the brightness control until a light background just begins to appear on the screen.

3. Adjust the contrast according to the gray-scale bar.

4. Adjust the overall gain until the major portion of the screen is optimally saturated (sonogram A).

5. Adjust the near gain so that the top area of the screen matches the area beneath it (sonogram B).

6. Adjust the far gain until echoes begin to appear on the bottom of the screen (sonogram F). Usually the far gain can be set at maximum.

Freeze Control

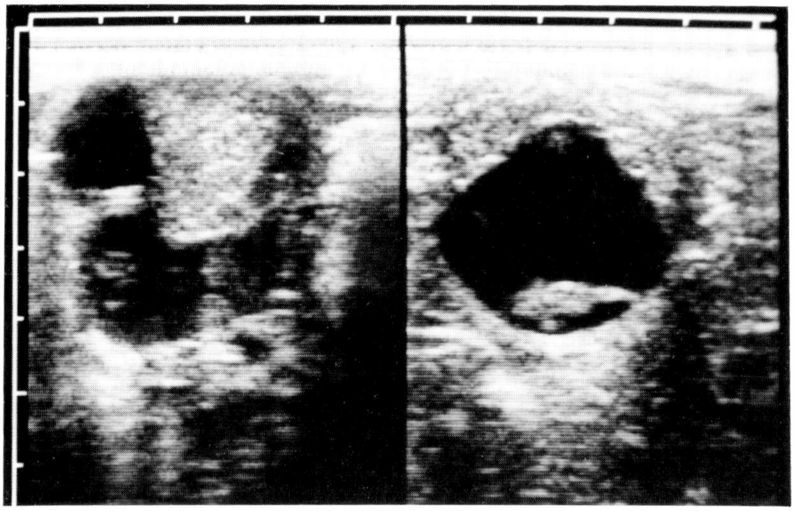

Side-by-side freezing of two images. The images are of a Day-29 corpus luteum and the corresponding embryonic vesicle. Modern scanners have a provision for freezing an image, allowing study or photography. The control button may be located on the console or in a remote box. We prefer to have the control button on the console because we normally have the console close to the operator and certainly within arm's length (pg 132); under these optimized circumstances, a remote control box can be a nuisance. Freezing is done through an image-storage function known as freeze-frame memory. In some scanners, especially the older models, the freeze-frame memory may involve only one sweep of beams across the transducer. Therefore, only every other scan line is seen and the resulting image is of low quality. This problem also may occur when attempting to freeze a videotaped image for detailed study or for still photography. In some scanners, several images may be frozen simultaneously and recalled as needed. The side-by-side provision on some scanners, shown above, allows the operator to freeze an image and then to continue scanning by means of an adjacent image. This provision is especially useful for comparing areas or to select the most desirable image for photography. In addition, a structure too wide for one screen can be photographed on two contiguous screens. The images from digital scan converters will remain in storage until released from the memory or until the scanner is turned off. However, images from analog scan converters begin to deteriorate slightly after approximately 10 minutes.

Checking Performance

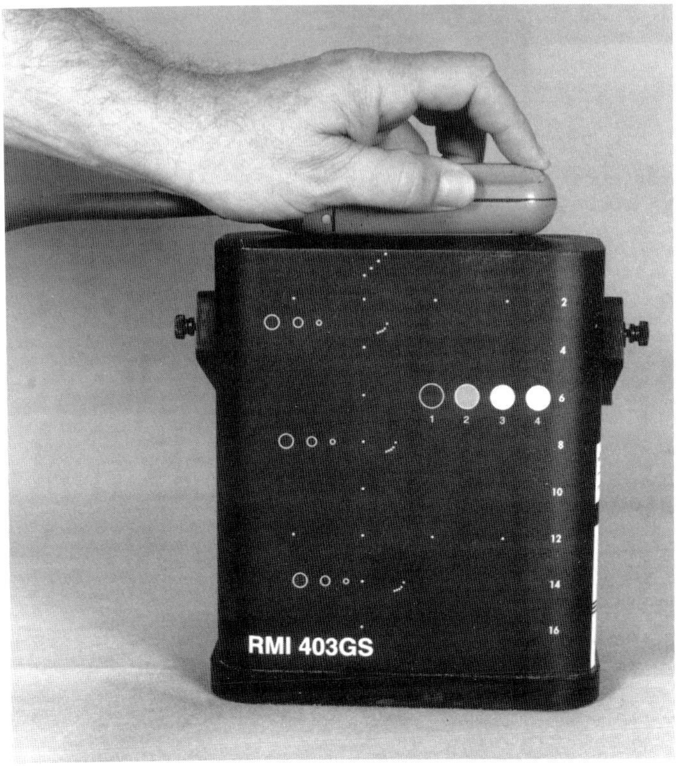

Tissue-mimicking testers or phantoms. This quality-assurance phantom was produced by Gammex RMI (source information: pg 195). Such devices can be used to monitor a scanner's continuing performance. The phantoms contain test objects (e.g., nylon filaments or pins, cylinders, cysts) embedded in tissue mimicking material (e.g., agar gel with dispersed and arranged carbon particles).

Quality assurance checks are useful because image degradation can occur gradually. In human medical hospitals, quality assurance checks are done at least annually. However, in the animal field, checks should be done more frequently. Portable animal scanners are subject to more rigorous conditions (e.g., dust, jolting, changing temperature and humidity) and animal sonographers may not have multiple scanners available for comparative purposes. When limited to one scanner, the sonographer is gradually conditioned to accept inferior quality without noticing a worsening problem.

Quality control programs have been described and reviewed in many publications *(e.g., 7, 25, 107)*. A sonographer's guide for establishing a quality assurance program for B-mode ultrasound imaging systems was produced recently by a maker of ultrasound phantoms (Gammex RMI; *137*) and is the source for many of the following notations. User's guides are also available with purchased phantoms.

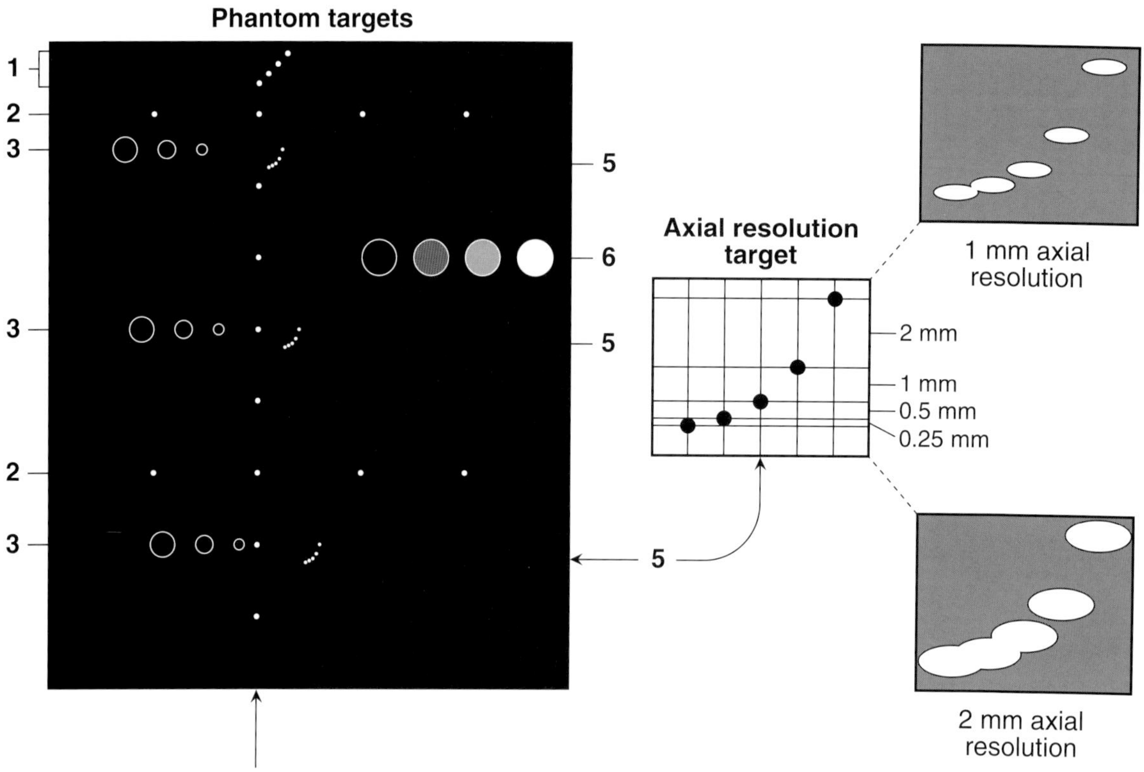

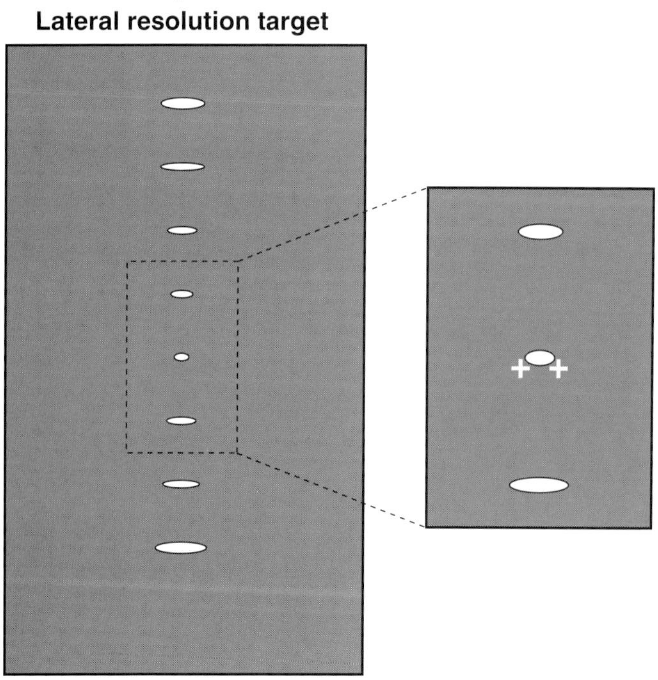

Key for phantom targets

1. Dead zone
2. Horizontal measurement
3. Cysts
4. Lateral resolution and vertical measurement
5. Axial resolution
6. Shade

Diagram of a quality-assurance phantom. For quality assurance, a baseline for each instrument (transducer and console) is established when it is new or at peak performance. The scanner, including the monitor, is adjusted to produce high-quality images from the phantom. The control settings (brightness, contrast, gain, focal zone) are recorded or marked so that subsequent tests can be directly compared. It is useful to produce hard copies of the phantom's images at baseline. A log of scanner performance data is usually kept in human hospitals, and some of the tests can be quantitated over time in graph form. Characteristics considered in quality tests include depth of penetration, linear measurement accuracy (horizontal and vertical distances), presence of artifacts, quality of cysts, and resolution (axial and lateral; pg 46). Depth of penetration may consider the deepest cyst of a given diameter that is barely visible. If the estimated penetration drops more than 1 cm, service is probably needed. Distance accuracy tests are easily performed by placing the cursors next to objects of known maximal distances, both vertical (Target 4) and horizontal (Target 2). Cysts (Target 3) should be anechoic and round when viewed in cross-section, and specular reflectors should be clear. Lateral-resolution tests use a vertical row of pins (diameter, 0.1mm) as shown in the diagram (Target 4). Images of the pins mimic the shape and width of the ultrasound beam, and measurements of the pin images indicate the changing lateral resolution at various depths. This occurs because a reflector encompassed by a beam is perceived as an object as wide as the beam by the scanner (pg 46). Examples of lateral resolution are <3 mm for a 3.5 MHz probe, and <1.5 mm for a 5.0 MHz probe. Axial resolution may be tested by pins placed in a curve, with the pins separated by distances of 2, 1, 0.5, and 0.25 mm as shown in the diagram (Target 5). The anechoic area between adjacent pins should be sufficient to allow horizontal placement of a separating line without contacting a marker. The resolutions are 1.0 mm and 2 mm in the two diagramed examples. In general, axial resolution should be 1 mm or less for transducers greater than 4 MHz. The dead zone (Target 1) is the area of noninformation beneath the transducer face. It can be checked for changes from baseline by using the indicated 4 pins, which represent depths of 1, 4, 7, and 10 mm from the interface of the probe and phantom. Aberrant horizontal lines often indicate circuitry problems, and vertical lines may indicate defective elements in the transducer (pg 80). Poor electric contacts in the cables or circuit boards or outside electrical interference also will be evident on the images of the phantom.

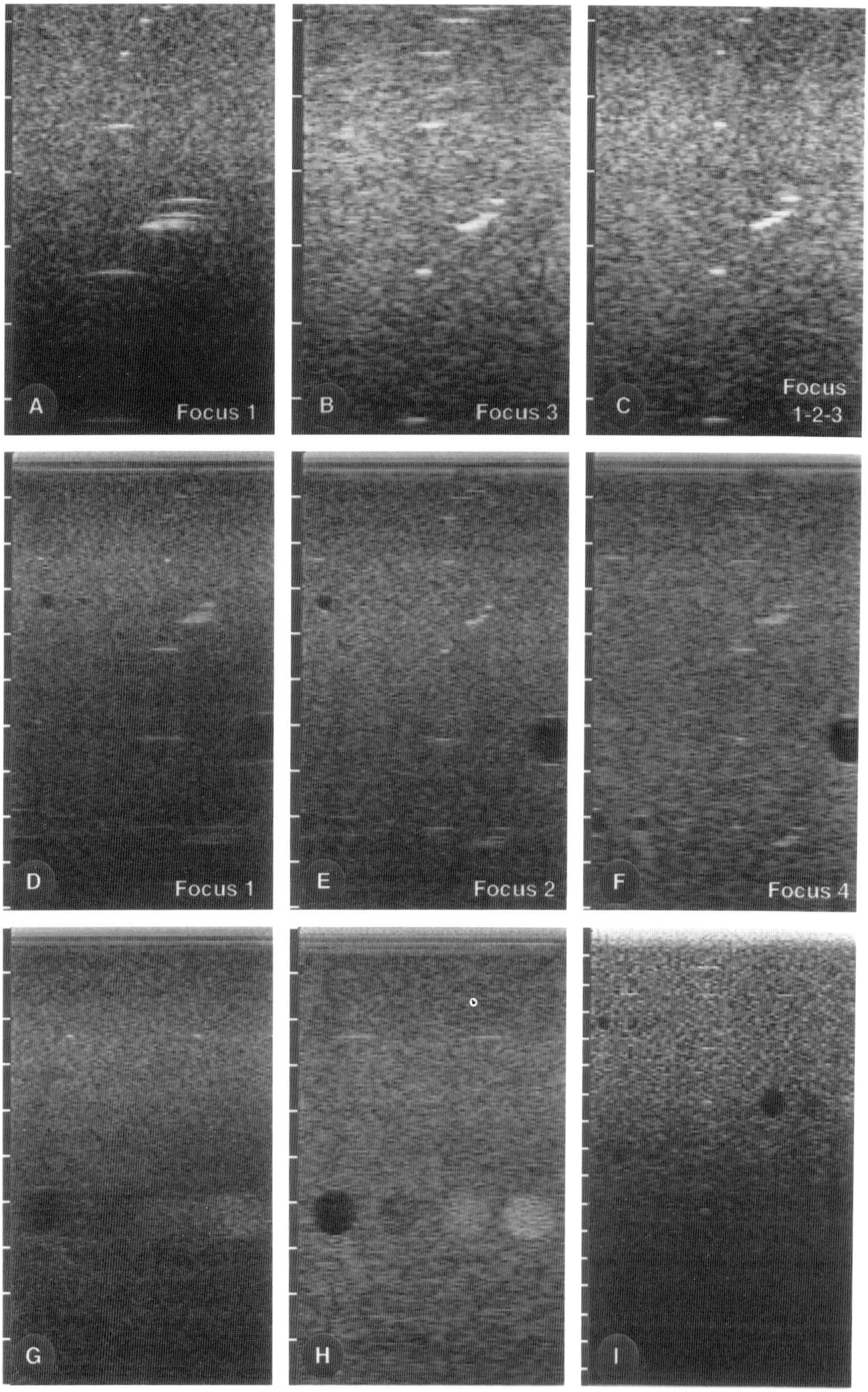
A
Focus 1
B
Focus 3
C
Focus
1-2-3
D
Focus 1
E
Focus 2
F
Focus 4
G
H
I

Images from a quality-assurance phantom (facing page). The scanner was an Aloka 500 (except for I), which has the multiple focusing provision. The phantom was described on previous pages. The placements of the 10 mm graduation marks and depth of penetration are functions of the transducer frequencies of 7.5 MHz (A, B, C), 5.0 MHz (D, E, F, G, H), and 3.5 MHz (I).

(A) The focal point at 13 mm is indicated by the smallest width of the vertical rows of 0.1 mm pins (Target 4). The changing lateral resolutions is indicated by the increasing width of the pins at depths of 23, 43, and 63 mm. The nearest axial resolution indicator (Target 5) is beyond the focal zone and not well imaged.

(B) The increased depth of the focal point (43 mm) demonstrates the effectiveness of the focal zone adjustment (Target 4). The axial resolution is in the focal zone (Target 5) and a better indicator than in image A. The separation of the pins indicates that the axial resolution is about 2 mm (pg 100).

(C) The combined focus adjustments produced an image equivalent to combined images A and B and, in addition, show improved lateral resolution at 23 mm because of the addition of focus 2.

(D) The focal point for focus 1 (Target 4) with the 5.0 MHz transducer is further (23 mm) than for focus 1 of the 7.5 MHz transducer (13 mm). The objects are less distinct because of the smaller imaged size as indicated by the closer graduation marks.

(E) The axial-resolution (Target 5) is better imaged because of the increased depth of the focal point (target 4).

(F) The 10 mm anechoic cyst (Target 6) is more distinct for focus 4 than for focuses 1 and 2. Even the 2 mm cyst is distinguishable at a depth of 80 mm. The axial resolution (Target 5) at 80 mm indicates a resolution of 2 mm.

(G, H) The echogenicity of the cysts at 60 mm is more distinct for focus 4 (H) than for focus 1 (G).

(I) The depth of penetration for this 3.5 MHz transducer is defective, as indicated by the near absence of information beyond approximately 100 mm.

Formalin-fixed tissue samples also are used to provide information on the imaging capabilities of selected tissues and boundaries *(7)*. Ultrasonic propagation through tissue fixed with 4% formalin and 5% potassium dichromate is similar to that in fresh tissue *(10)*. Ultrasound phantoms can be prepared also from intravenous fluid bags filled with liquid agar and appropriate objects *(see reference 154 for instructions)*; such phantoms are being used as teaching aids (e.g., demonstrating the origin of artifacts and handling ultrasonically guided instruments).

Scanners Used in Human Medicine

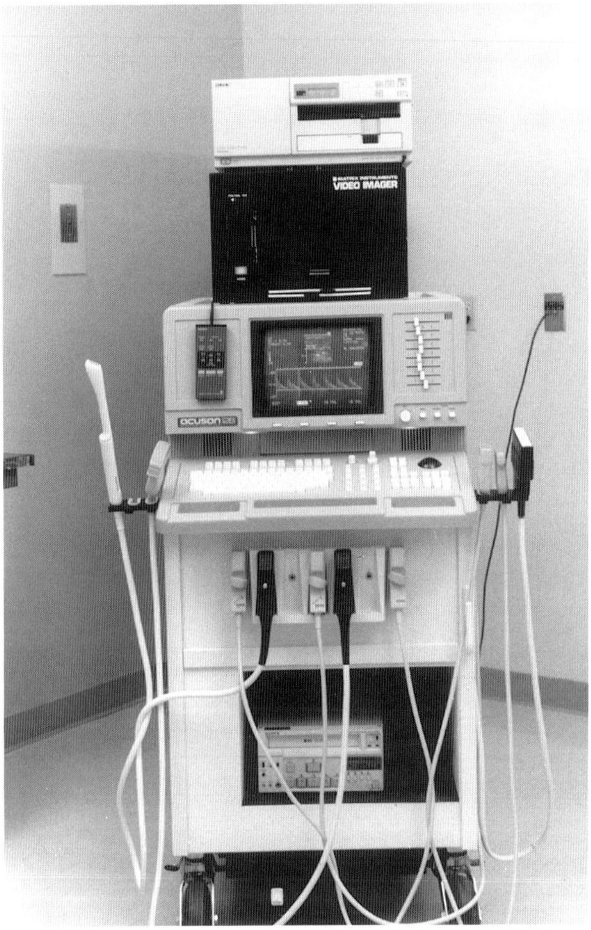

Acuson 128XP. Several makes of multipurpose scanners are in use in human medicine. Such scanners are at the forefront of the ultrasound technology. Even though financially prohibitive (e.g., $250,000) and not meeting some animal requirements, they are harbingers of the capabilities that eventually may be available for animal use. The Acuson computed sonography system displays information in several operating modes: 1) 2-D imaging (B-mode), 2) spectral Doppler (blood flow monitoring), 3) color Doppler (real-time spatial visualization of blood flow), and 4) M-mode (graphically shows changes over time, such as fetal cardiac function and chamber dimensions). All the transducer imaging formats or arrays shown elsewhere (pg 38) are incorporated (linear, sector, curved, phased). The transducer on the left side of the rack is a transvaginal or endovaginal transducer that is commonly used for examining the internal reproductive organs of women. Multiple focal zones can be selected and are indicated by carets on the graduated depth scale. These features are now becoming available in veterinary scanners (e.g., multiple transducer frequencies, Pie Medical and Ausonics; multiple focal points, Aloka and Pie Medical). Gain is controlled in several ways and features a depth-gain-compensation provision under the control of the eight sliding levers to the right of the viewing screen. A curve indicating the gain settings can be displayed on the images as shown on the following sonograms. It also has a provision for adjusting frame rate. Apparently, a slower rate may sometimes help eliminate reverberation artifacts. Other features are shown in the following sonograms.

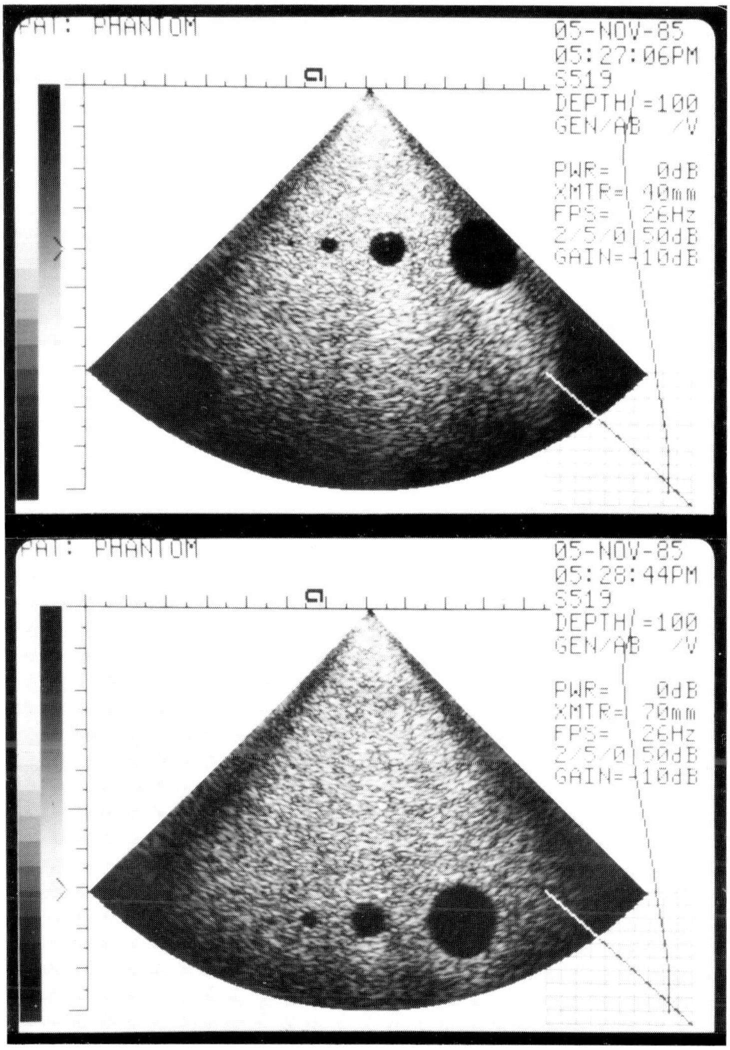

Images of an ultrasound phantom taken with an Acuson 128. A 5.0 MHz, phased-array, sector transducer was used to produce the images. The phantom is the same one used with a veterinary scanner for producing the images shown elsewhere (pg 63, pg 95; compare the resolutions). The fluid-filled objects are 2, 5, 10, and 20 mm in diameter. The Acuson 128 has a control for varying the focal depth. Settings of 4 cm and 7 cm were used for the images on the top and bottom, respectively, as indicated by the arrowheads on the centimeter scale. The values for several variables are automatically displayed (upper right). The curved vertical line on the right represents the gain-control settings for various depths. Note the sharp outlines of the fluid-filled objects and the near-absence of artifactual echoes within the fluid.

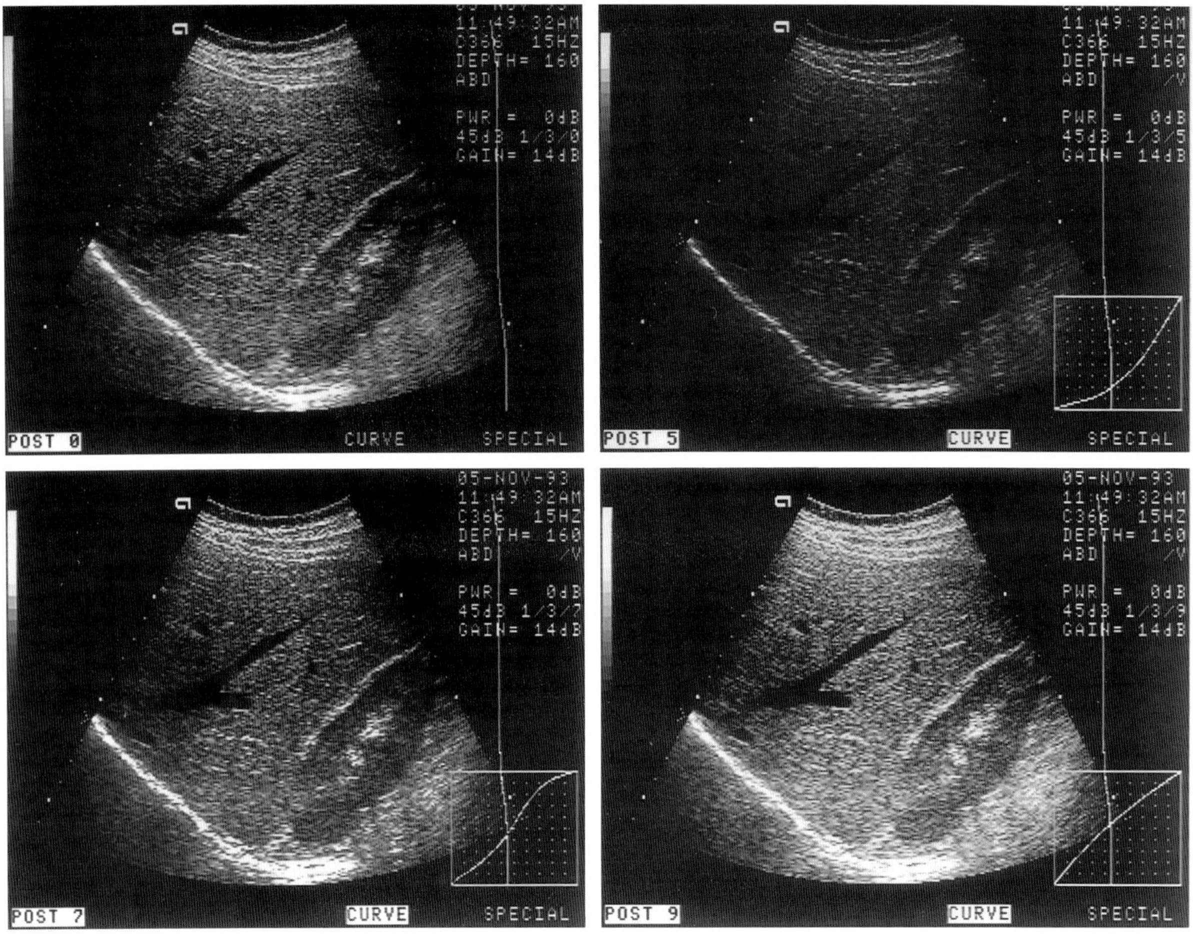

Postprocessing curves. The sonograms were taken of a liver and kidney with a curved-array transducer. A postprocessing curve (pg 53) is displayed on three of the images to define the relationships between echo amplitude and the selected pixel intensity. The programmed settings are indicated (lower left) and the curves depicting the settings are shown on the lower right. A straight line (not shown) depicts a linear relationship between echo amplitude and screen brightness; no gray levels are suppressed. At least one recently introduced veterinary scanner has what is apparently a similar provision and is called the gamma curve (Pie Medical; source information: pg 193). This provision was described recently (*J. Equine Vet. Sci, 14:475-47, 1994*). Adjustment of the gamma curve can be used to enhance a specific group of gray-scale signals for compatibility with the echotexture of a given tissue or organ. For example, the middle level of the gray scale can be enhanced to display the subtle tissue changes of the liver.

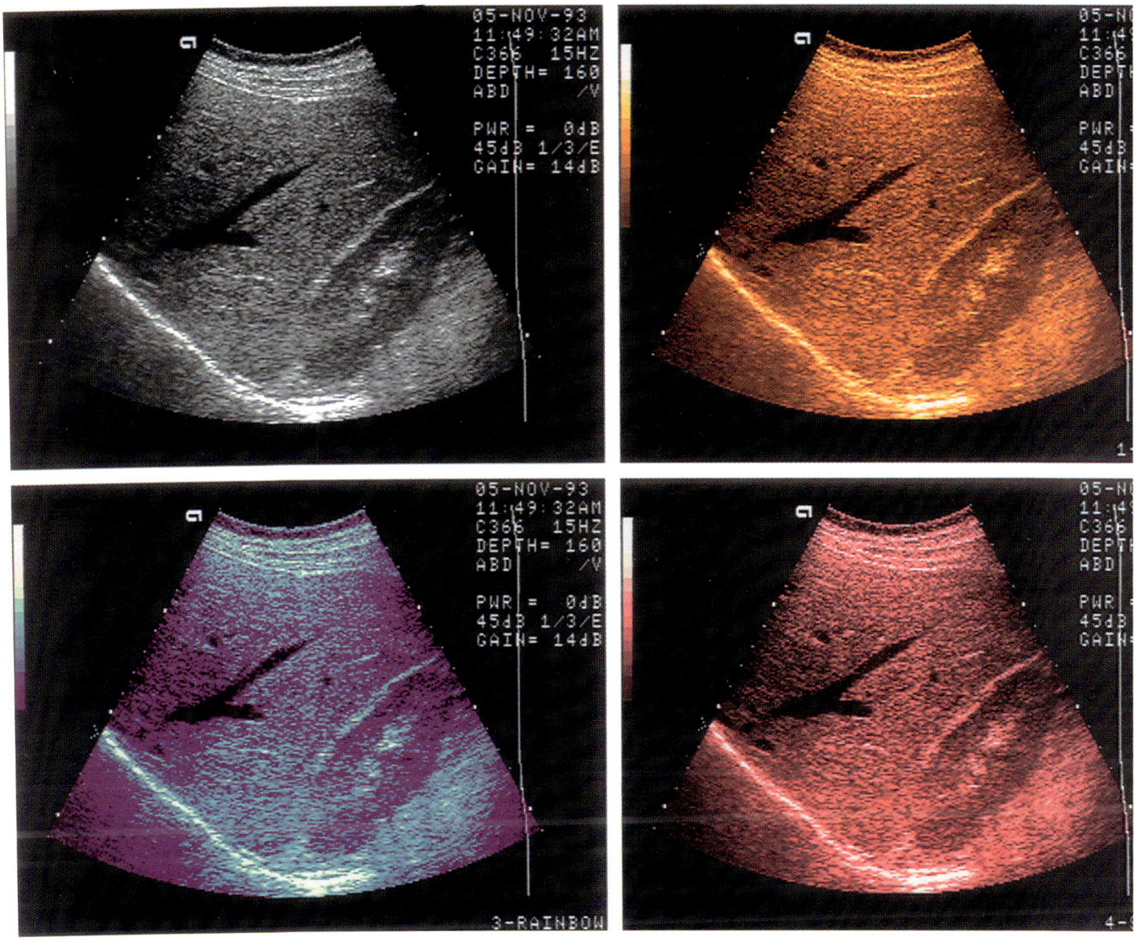

Colorized sonograms. The sonograms depict colorization of liver-kidney images. The images are from an Acuson 128XP, and the sonograms were made with a Sony videographic printer. Colorization is favored by some sonographers but apparently is not used by others. A newly introduced capability is the colorization of a perfusion (e.g., for renal studies). The colorization can be compared to the conventional gray-scale display on the facing page.

Colorization also has been used in recent years to depict various shades of gray in different colors. This feature is one of the capabilities of an auxiliary system being marketed for animal studies by Corometrics (Medimage; pg 125)

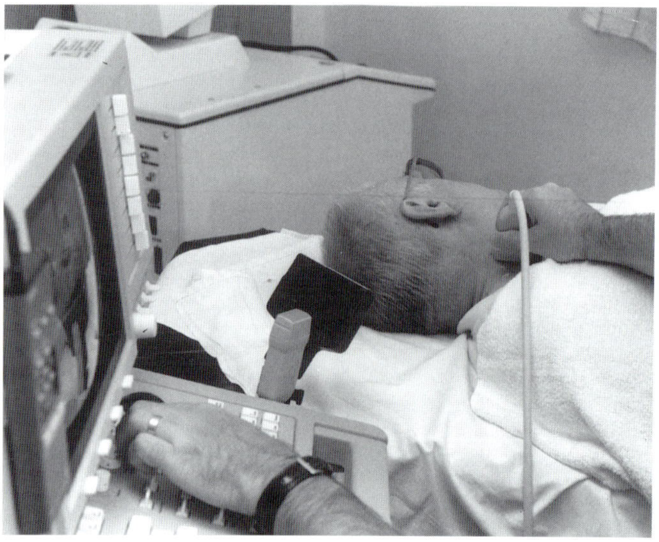

Linear-array transducer applied to the neck. This transducer placement was used to produce the Doppler sonograms shown below.

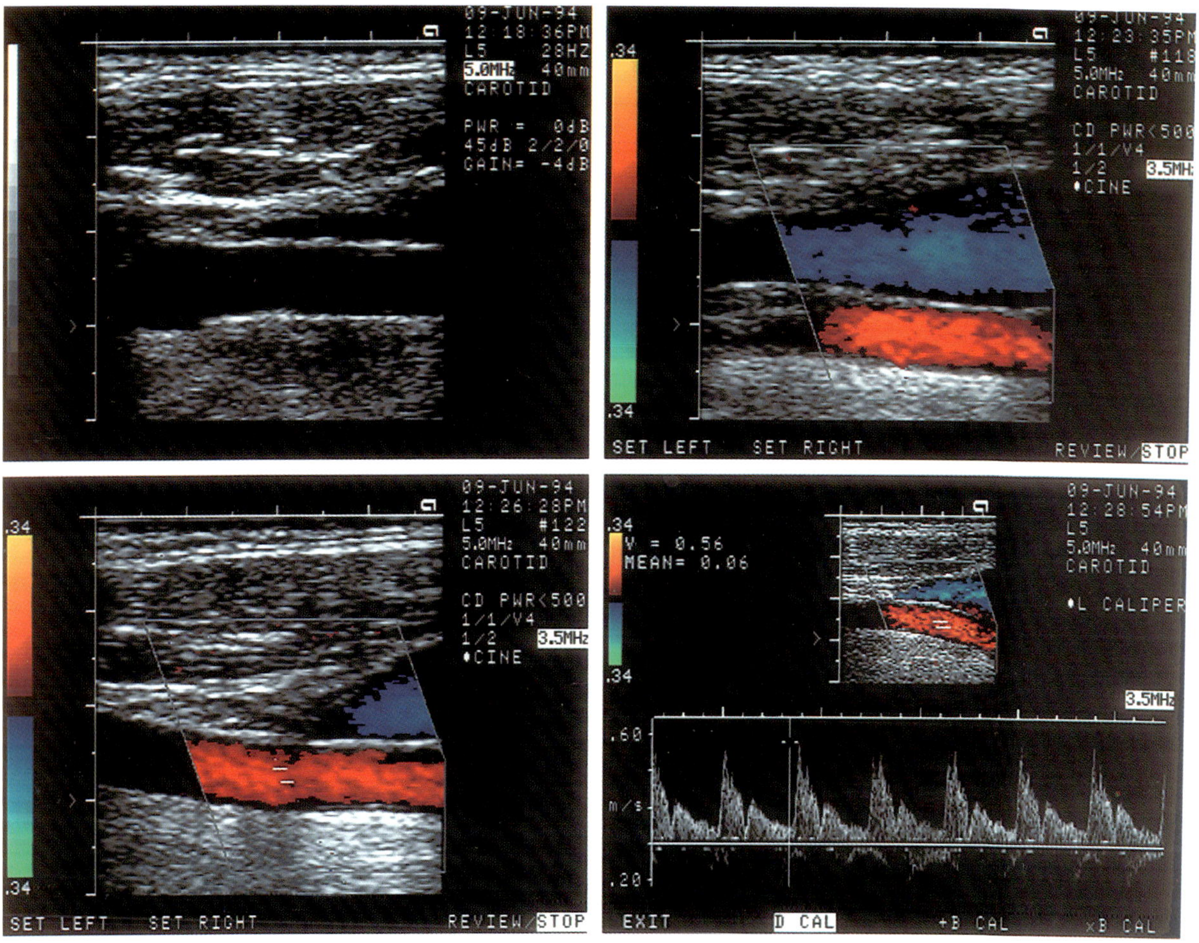

Doppler assessment of blood vessels (facing page).

Upper left: Sonogram showing the echogenic borders of the carotid artery.

Upper right: Doppler mode depicting blood flow in the carotid artery (red) and jugular vein (blue).

Lower left: A sampling cursor or gate has been superimposed on the carotid for assessment of blood velocity (meters/sec) in the sampled area

Lower right: The velocity is displayed on the image readout as related to the location of the cursor on the apex of a wave.

Doppler techniques have been used for many years for studies in humans *(50, 160)*. A review of Doppler imaging for functional assessment of early uteroplacental and fetoplacental circulations in humans apparently will be published in the January 1995 issue of Theriogenology. Doppler techniques are in their inception for studies of blood flow to the reproductive organs of animals. The dynamic vascular system of the internal genitalia of cattle during the estrous cycle has been studied by the Doppler approach *(168)*. Apparently, Doppler studies have begun on the blood flow of the umbilical cord in horses *(108)*.

At the present time, scanners in the conventional veterinary market apparently do not have the color Doppler provision. A color Doppler for flow mapping that is being used in small animals, but apparently has not yet been used for animal reproduction work, is available for approximately $50,000 (source information: pg 194). Used scanners with color Doppler capabilities can be obtained for $30,000 to $60,000 (inquire to distributors listed in appendix; pg 191).

Spectral Dopplers (those designed to give velocity readings) are available in pulsed-wave and continuous-wave formats. In the pulsed-wave format, the same crystals are used for both sending and receiving as in conventional B-mode scanners (pg 37). The continuous-wave format, however, has a different set of crystals for sending and receiving and therefore has greater penetrability and can determine higher blood velocities. A spectral Doppler (no color) currently being used for small animals can be obtained for approximately $26,000 (source information: pg 194).

Selecting a Make and Model

Points to ponder in selecting a scanner.

1. General
   A. Linear-array versus sector transducers (pg 38)
   B. Transducer and cable design (pg 86)
   C. Transducer frequency (pg 88)
   D. Portability (pg 93)
   E. Annotation and labeling provisions (pg 94)
   F. Measuring provisions (pg 94)
   G. Freeze frame memory provisions and quality (pg 98, pg 118)
   H. Zoom and magnification provisions and quality (pg 111)
   I. Photography and videotaping provisions (Chapter 7)
   J. Battery power-pack option (pg 111)

2. Quality of images
   A. Specifications
      1) Number of elements (pg 41)
      2) Frame rate (pg 45, pg 104)
      3) Focusing methods (pg 47); multiple focal points desirable (pg 40)
      4) Number of shades of gray (pg 55)

   B. Results of personal trial
      1) Images smooth, pleasant, and not checkered
      2) Able to meet specific needs. Examples:
         a) Detect mature corpus luteum
         b) Detect small follicles (e.g., 3 mm)
         c) Detect small embryonic vesicles

3. Durability and reliability of scanner

4. Longevity and service record of the company

5. Suitability for other uses

The purchase of an ultrasound scanner is a major investment (e.g., $16,000), so potential buyers are justified in thoroughly researching the purchase. Veterinary ultrasonography continues to be a volatile marketing area. There have been several turnovers in companies or marketing lines, and technological changes are frequent. This chapter, as well as most chapters, contains information that should be useful in deciding whether to purchase a scanner and in selecting the most appropriate make, model, and options. References to appropriate pages are noted in the above list. Because of the magnitude of the investment, prospective buyers should expect to have scanners demonstrated to them, preferably on site. This approach, combined with consultations with experienced colleagues and study of published information, should enable a potential buyer to make reasonable decisions.

Makes and models of scanners vary widely in capabilities and incidental provisions, as listed above under Topic 1. All individuals will desire high quality and good service, for example, but may differ in their general needs. This is especially true for clinical versus research requirements. Researchers may want elaborate provisions for annotations, measurement (e.g., area), photography and videotaping, and multiple freeze-frame memories. Clinicians may prefer less elaborate schemes, especially if it means a lower price and fewer breakdowns. Provisions should be consistent with the needs—neither inadequate nor excessive.

Some scanners have zoom controls to enlarge a selected area or magnification controls to enlarge the entire image. However, the resulting images may be poor, especially if the pixels (pg 56) become so large that they are visible. Postprocessing magnification of a portion (zoom control) or all (magnification control) of an image in such scanners may provide no real improvement in resolution—just an increase in size. Other scanners may use all or most of the pixels on the screen when providing an enlarged area; therefore, truly increasing resolution. In regard to linear-array versus sector systems, it should be noted that some scanners can be used with either type of transducer. We prefer the linear-array system for intrarectal imaging the reproductive tract because of the full width of view near the transducer (pg 38). The battery option may be crucial for some situations. Currently available battery models (source information: pg 191) include the Ultra-scan II (Alliance Medical; *156*) and SonoAce 88P (Medison America).

The expected image quality (Topic 2 in the above list) should take into account the scanner's specifications, especially with regard to meeting certain minimums. A scanner should not, however, be selected on the basis of its specifications alone. For example, a scanner with many elements will provide poor quality if other aspects of the engineering (e.g., damping, electrical insulation) are poor. Good resolving power and penetrating capability are not assured on the basis of transducer frequency. Many other factors are involved. The most reliable information on quality is obtained from a personal trial under the potential buyer's conditions. Ideally, a potential buyer should learn first what a good image looks like by observing images on scanners owned by experienced colleagues or scientists. Ultrasonographers in human medicine also may be conveniently available for this purpose. A buyer should require that the images are smooth, pleasant, and free from the obnoxious checkered appearance of large pixels (pg 56). Buyers can prepare a list of needs and then determine by trial whether the scanner performs as desired. An excellent criterion for evaluating the quality of a scanner centers around its ability to consistently image a developing or mature corpus luteum. For example, select several horses with known date and side of ovulation. The mares should not exceed Day 10, because the corpus luteum may become undetectable in an occasional mare after Day 10. The buyer then can test the ability of the scanner to consistently present a clear and sharp image of the corpus luteum. Poor scanners, even those with a 5.0 MHz transducer, will fail the test.

Topics 3 and 4 in the above list concern the durability of the scanner and the reliability and speed of the repair service. Ultrasound scanners are highly specialized instruments and local repair service usually will not be available. In this regard, however, local repair shops might be found that can handle minor problems such as power-cord defects, thereby eliminating shipment costs. Consultation with owners and users is probably the best way to obtain information on the relative durability of the model and the service record of the distributor. The selection of a scanner for transrectal use also may include consideration of other possible uses (Topic 5). Scanners are being adapted for use in many species and body systems. Other clinical applications include diagnosing and monitoring the following: 1) urinary bladder calculi and other diseases, 2) aortic aneurysms, 3) heart diseases, 4) abdominal problems such as biliary and renal calculi, ascites, and neoplasia, 5) joint and tendon problems, and 6) eye or orbital diseases or injuries. If a scanner is to be used for purposes other than imaging the reproductive tract, sector transducers or systems that are compatible with both sector and linear-array transducers may have advantages.

Chapter 7

HARD COPY

Hard copy is defined as the readable printed copy from a machine, such as a computer. In ultrasonography, the term is commonly used for photographs (ultrasonograms) or videotapes of images. Communication and documentation of results are important aspects of ultrasonography. Specialized instruments and knowledge are required to produce high-quality hard copy, whether a Polaroid image for an owner's scrapbook or a set of images for a professional or scientific publication. The preparation of projection slides and videotapes is useful for educational and communicational purposes, both for the clinician and researcher. Scientific or lay articles on research or clinical reports involving ultrasound depend on the photographic skills of the ultrasonographer and the publisher. It is depressing to produce high-quality images only to have much of the quality and definition lost in the production of hard copy. It is even more depressing to succeed in producing a high-quality photograph only to have much of its quality lost during duplication in a publication.

Hard-copy technologies are extensive and changing rapidly. This chapter describes the instruments and techniques commonly used in ultrasonography for recording and storing images. The chapter represents an updating of a chapter prepared by R. A. Pierson for the original book *(58)*. Attention is given to the following: 1) Polaroid photography; 2) negative-based photography; 3) preparation of slides for projection; 4) production of videotapes and preparation of photographs from videotapes, and 5) preparation of slides and photographs with the aid of a computer. In the production of photographs, a freeze-frame memory in the scanner or a frame-grabber in a computer are used. The quality of the photographs therefore depends upon the quality of the real-time images and the quality of the freeze-frame provision, as well as on the quality of photographic instrumentation and technique. Integration of scanners, tape recorders, and personal computers is a recent and rapidly advancing technology. Preparation of hard copy from such integration is discussed. Some of the information in this chapter was obtained from a review of display and recording devices for ultrasonography *(106)*.

Polaroid Photography

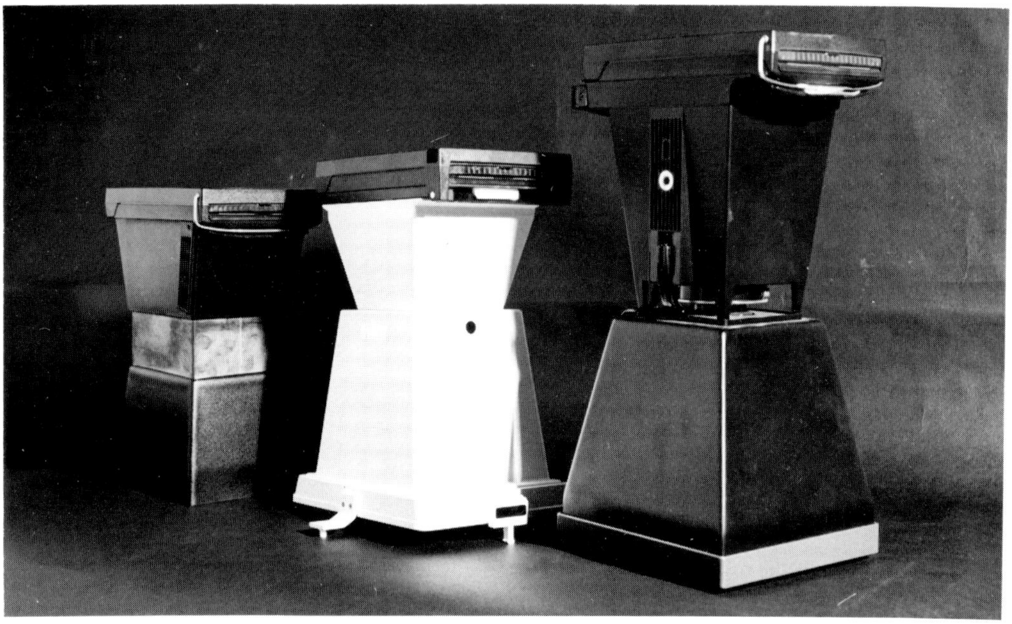

Examples of Polaroid cameras used with animal ultrasound systems. In some systems, the camera shroud is hand-held over the viewing screen; in others, the shroud is hinged and provides a stable support for the camera. Polaroid film is much more expensive than negative-based film, resulting in high running costs for the Polaroid system. In this regard, at least one scanner used for transrectal imaging of animal reproductive tracts has a left-to-right switching mechanism so that two images can be recorded on one film. This provision reduces the photographic costs. Polaroid photography provides almost immediate viewing of the images. This is advantageous in practice situations and in some research applications. Polaroid images are also an effective way of backing up other photographic systems, when it is essential that a record of the ultrasound scan not be lost.

Unexposed Polaroid films have a shelf-life of approximately nine months at room temperature. The processing chemistry integral to instant film is the limiting factor in storing the film. Freezing Polaroid films will not appreciably extend the life of the film. Archival qualities of developed Polaroid film depend upon storage conditions. If images are stored in acid-free paper under controlled temperature, light, and humidity, they should last indefinitely. However, if stored in traditional paper files, the life of the print may not exceed five years. Prints exposed to light and fluctuations in temperature and humidity will fade appreciably within the first year, although some Polaroid films may be coated to increase the archival qualities of the print.

Film types 611 and 667 were designed for photographing gray-scale images and provide 3.25 x 4.25 inch photographs. Type 611 provides extended gray-scale information but is more difficult to use because it has no effective ISO (film-speed) rating. Shutter-speed and aperture adjustments are made from basic recommendations for exposure, included with the film. Settings depend on the type of viewing screen and brightness and contrast settings. The camera controls are adjusted from the initial recommendation according to the ultrasonographer's interpretation of the gray scale. Film type 667 is higher in contrast and is rated at 3000 ISO. The short exposure times with this film are advantageous in systems in which the camera shroud is hand-held against the viewing screen or when there is a likelihood of vibrations in the camera-scanner complex. In the past year, Polapan 400 has become available. It provides medium contrast and a 4 x 5 inch format.

Technical questions about specific applications and characteristics of Polaroid films may be addressed to Polaroid Resource Center at (800) 225-1618.

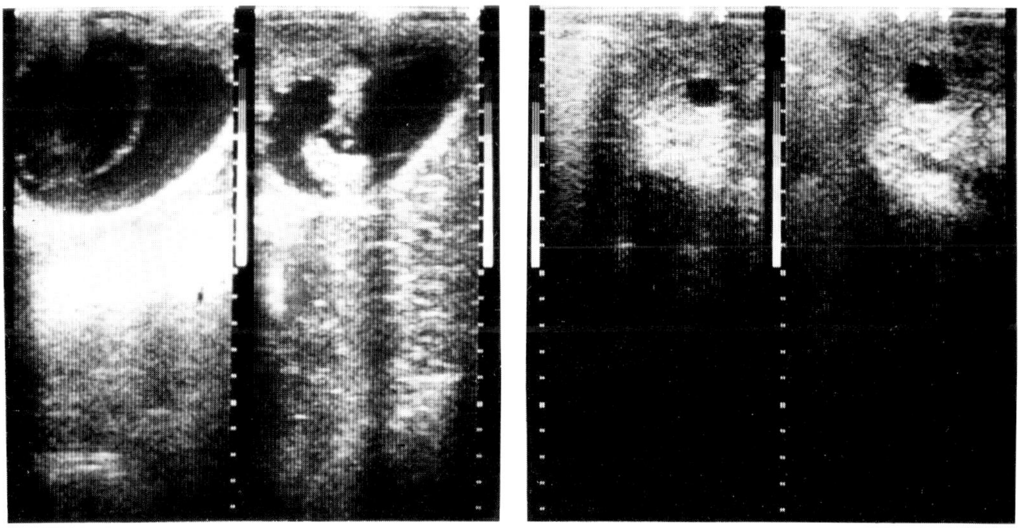

Sequential Polaroid photographs made by using a switching mechanism on the ultrasound scanner for photographing two images on one film. The pair of sonograms on the left are of Day-48 unilaterally fixed equine twins. The pair of sonograms on the right are of Day-14 and Day-15 twin embryonic vesicles.

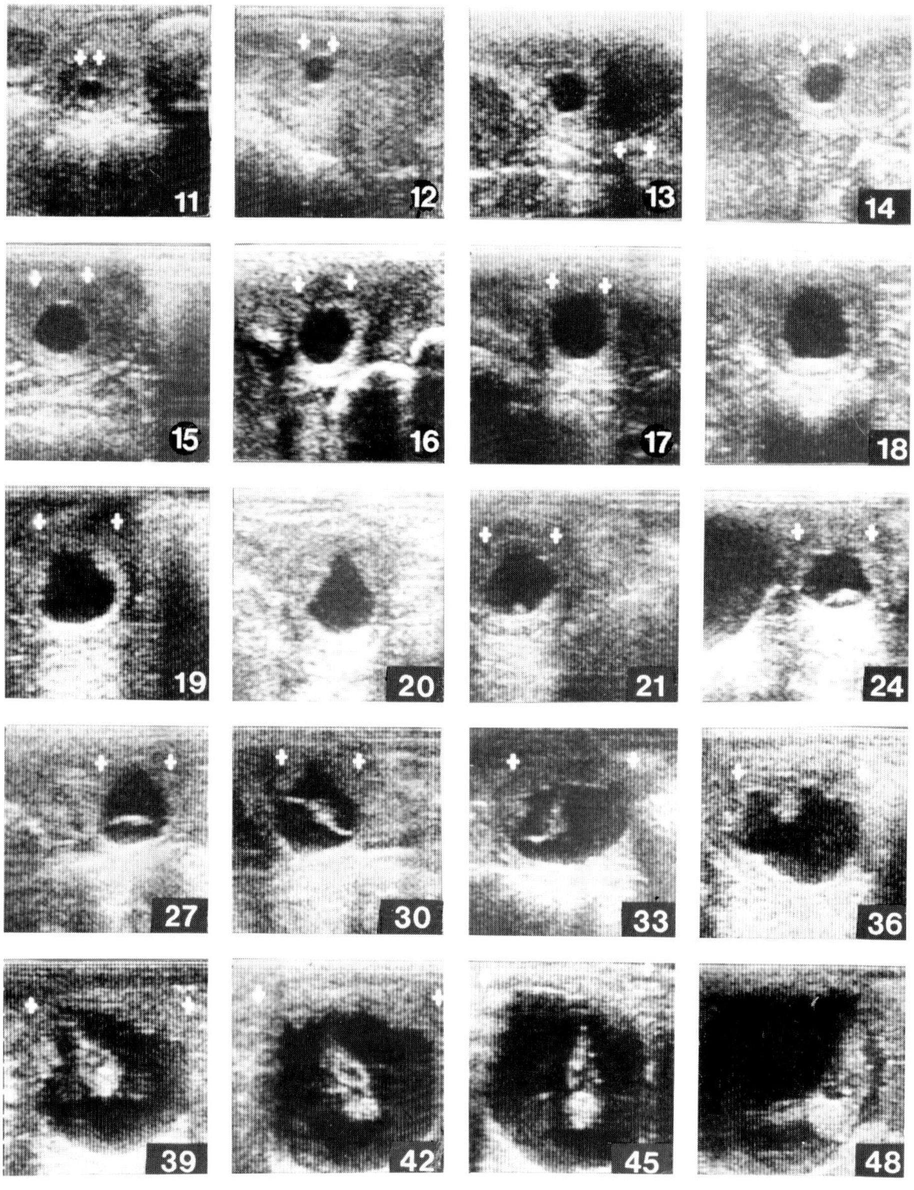

A series of cropped Polaroid photographs, showing the sequential changes in ultrasonic anatomy of the early conceptus. The number in the lower-right corner is the number of days from ovulation. This series is of historical interest; it represents the original detailed study of the changing ultrasonic anatomy of the early equine conceptus *(51)*. Film type 667 was used.

Negative-Based Photography

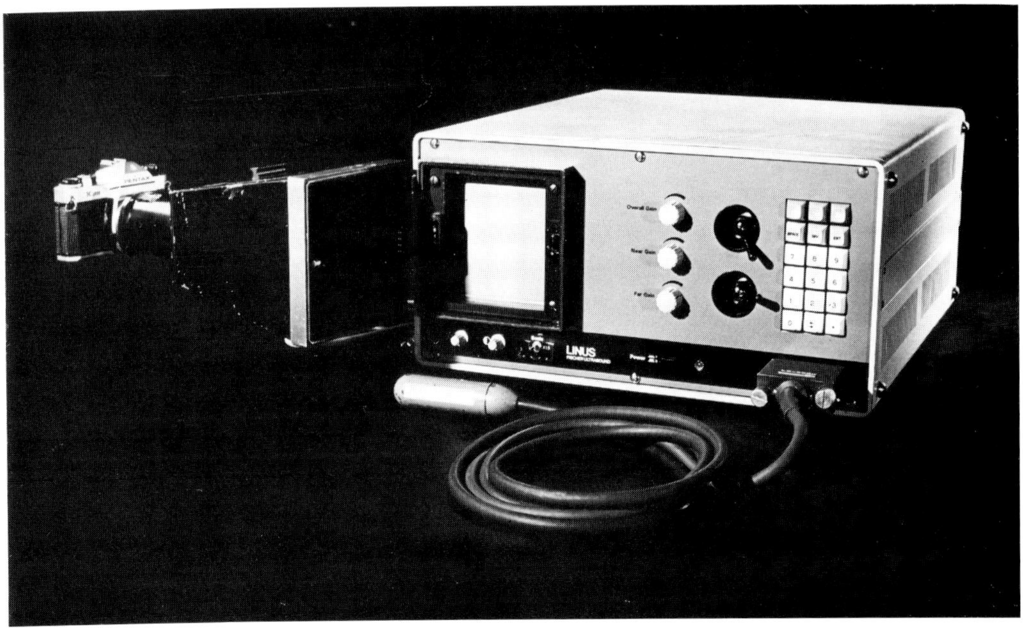

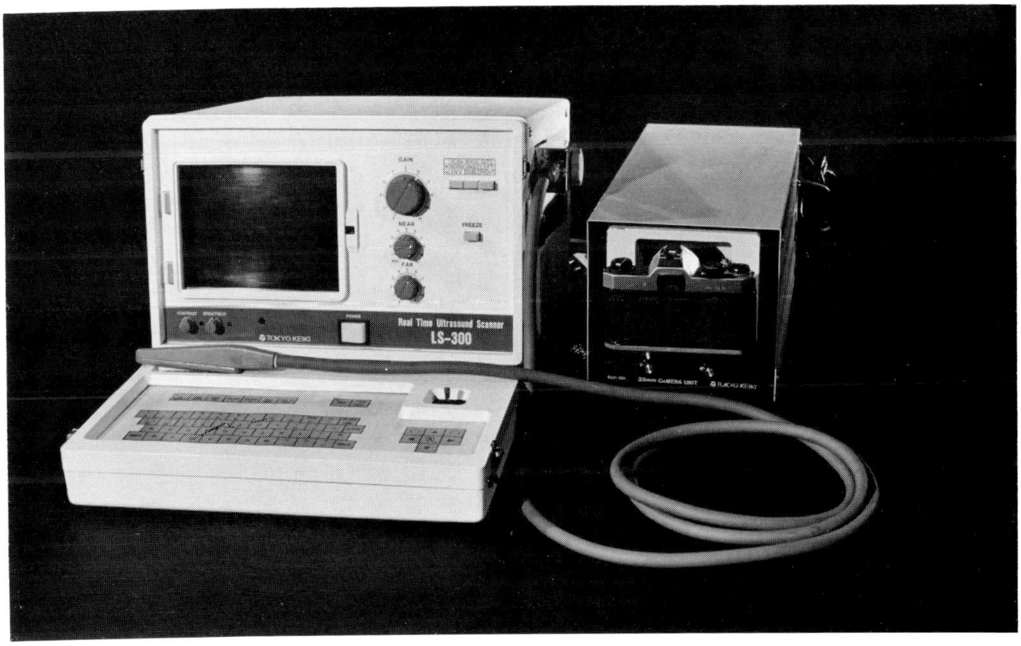

Examples of customized 35 mm camera systems. In one system, the camera is fitted to a shroud that attaches to the scanner as in some Polaroid systems. The shroud is closed and an exposure made. The camera and shroud may be removed or swung away from the screen on its mounting hinges. The second system is an enclosed auxiliary arrangement, consisting of a high-resolution six-inch television monitor, close-focusing lens, and camera body. This system is attached to the ultrasound scanner through video connections and acts as a slave monitor. In both systems, the desired image must be "frozen" on the ultrasound viewing screen before the exposures are made. In scanners with multiple freeze-frame memories, side-by-side images can be taken with one exposure. Both systems provide high-quality hard copy. The auxiliary system is more suited to research needs or centralized examining areas.

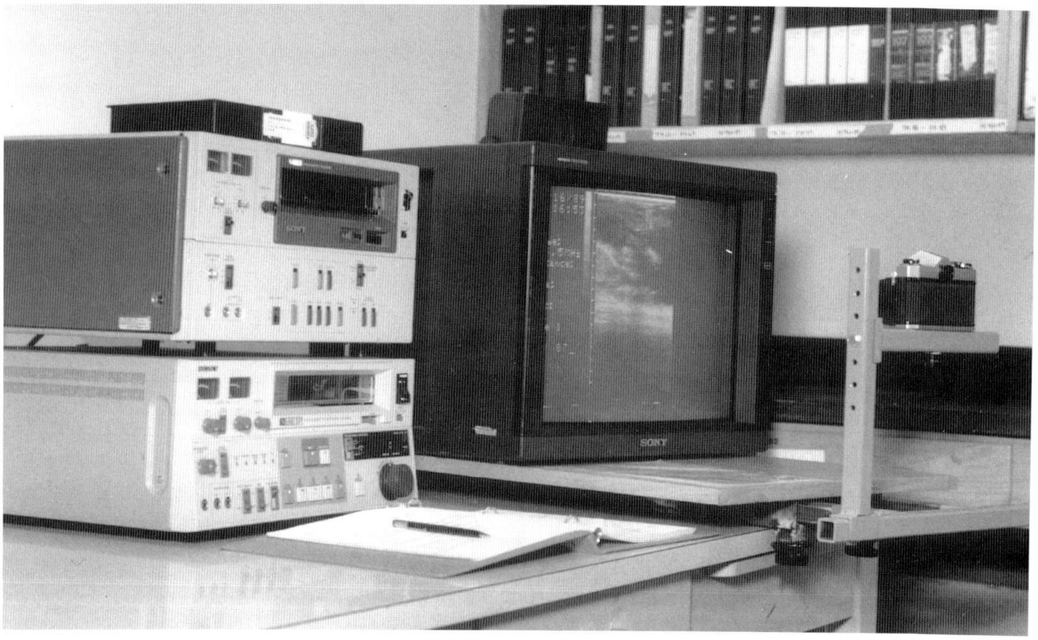

Preparing photographs from a TV monitor. A 35 mm camera is mounted on an adjustable stand. This system is used for direct photography when the information has been stored on videotape. It provides greater flexibility than when photographs are taken off the ultrasound screen as described above. This system provides excellent quality prints.

In our laboratory, the record-keeping system involves an entry onto a photographic record sheet as each exposure is made. There is a separate line for each exposure and a separate page for each roll of film. Thus, each exposure is identified with animal number, project, date, and general description. Depending on the data display or annotation capabilities of the ultrasound scanner, each negative contains specific information that uniquely identifies it and may be used to cross reference the description in the log book. After film processing, the negatives are placed in transparent polyethylene sheets that hold an entire roll of 36 exposures (Print File Archival Negative Preservers, Photo Plastic Products, Orlando, FL). Contact sheets, which display all images on the film roll on one 8 x 10-inch sheet of photographic paper, may be made without removing the negatives from the holder. The log sheets, negatives, and contact sheets are stored in three-ring binders for easy reference. When desired, selected images may be photographically enlarged for further study or publication. Individual ultrasound images may be viewed as contact-size or enlarged prints. For display purposes, we have enlarged some images to 16 x 20 inches, with excellent results.

Many emulsions currently available in 35 mm film can record the range of gray-scale shades used in ultrasonography. More than a cursory description of 35 mm films is beyond the scope of this text. Detailed descriptions of films and their individual characteristics are available in the photographic literature.

It is our current practice to photographically record ultrasound images on T-MAX 100 film (Eastman Kodak, Rochester, NY). This film appears to give accurate rendition of the gray shades encountered in our use of ultrasound. It is rated at ISO 100, which, with our systems, allows us to use a medium aperture with a reasonably fast shutter speed (for example, f5.6 at 1/2 second). This is important because the central portion of most lenses is sharper than the edge, and smaller apertures improve depth of field, helping to compensate for small focusing errors. Longer exposures may result in blurring, especially if the stand for the camera-ultrasound complex is attached to the restraining chute or if the source of the image is videotape freeze-frame where there is potential for jitter. The T-MAX 100 film has excellent resolving power and extremely fine grain, allowing a high degree of enlargement. For this and the above considerations, use of slower, fine-grain films is not recommended, especially in barns. Faster films (e.g., Kodak Tri-X and T-MAX 400, both ISO 400) are also available. Owing to its finer grain, T-MAX 400 should supplant Tri-X where shorter exposures or higher f-ratios are required.

Technical questions about Kodak films may be answered by contacting Kodak Technical Service (800) 242-2424.

Other Copy Methods

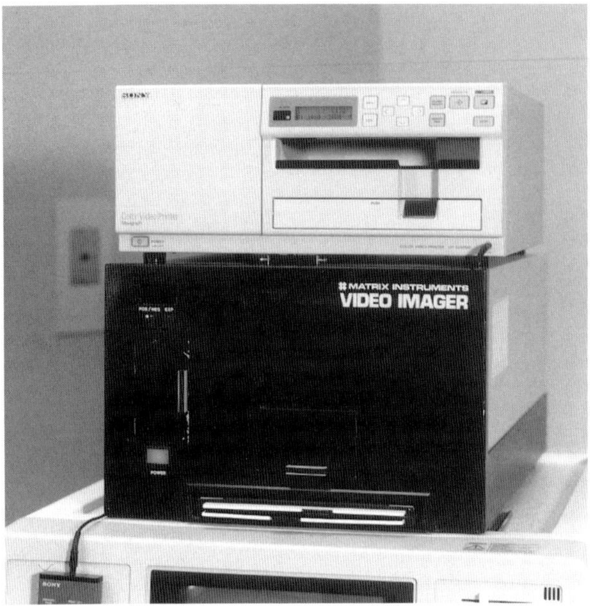

A video printer (upper) and a multiformat camera (lower). In recent years, video printers have become available for the immediate production of high-quality prints. The printing heads contain minute heating elements that imprint approximately 6 to 9 dots per mm. In the Sony 3000 to 5000 series, the input video signal is digitally processed in frame memory, so that 1 to 4 images can be printed on one sheet. It takes about 80 seconds to output a 140 x 100 mm print. More than 500 TV lines of horizontal resolution are obtained, involving 716 x 468 pixels. The printers produced by the Sony Corporation cost a few thousand dollars but provide publication-quality prints in black-and-white or color. Examples of photographs produced with a Sony video printer (UP-3000) are shown elsewhere (pg 106, pg 108).

For black-and-white prints of ultrasonograms, a quality thermal video printer can be obtained for less than $1,000 (e.g., Sony UP-870MD, Mitsubishi P50U). Furthermore, the cost of the thermally sensitized paper is minimal (8 to 10¢ per print for the Sony 870). The Sony units can be connected to either the scanner or a videotape machine. Print-out time also is minimal (approximately 4 seconds). Apparently the archival qualities of the paper have not been determined. The black-and-white thermal printers are very compatible with ultrasound scanners and are available from distributors of ultrasound scanners and supplies (source information: pg 191).

Multiformat cameras record high-quality images, but they must be viewed with transmitted light as are X-ray films. This system is commonly used in hospitals equipped with X-ray viewing screens and by operators accustomed to viewing X-ray films. Some examples of multiformat cameras are those made by Dunn, Schiff, and Matrix instrument companies. Prices vary from $7,000 to $15,000, depending on individual specifications, such as single format (fixed-lens system) or multiformat (lens system changes to fit several formats). Images are sent to the camera through video connections (digital scan converters) or XYZ connections (analog scan converters) and are recorded on 8 x 10-inch X-ray film. Commonly, 4, 6, 9, or 25 images are placed on one sheet. The size of an image is approximately 4 x 5 inches for the four-on-one format and approximately the size of a 35 mm slide for the 25-on-one format.

Projection Slides

Projection slides of ultrasound images can be prepared in many ways, including the following:

1) Ektachrome ER or EPR slide film (Eastman Kodak, Rochester, NY) may be used directly in the camera system.
2) Photographic prints prepared from negatives may be rephotographed using a copy stand and tungsten-balanced Ektachrome EPY or EPT slide film (Eastman Kodak).
3) Pan-X film may be used in the camera system and developed with a reverse processing kit available through Kodak product distributors.
4) Photographic negatives may be temporarily mounted in slide holders and rephotographed using a slide duplicator and negative film. The result is a positive image suitable for projection.
5) A 35 mm instant-slide system manufactured by Polaroid Corporation may be used. The entire roll of slide film is developed—in only a few minutes—with a separate processing kit.
6) Computer-generated slides of ultrasound images can be produced conveniently if an integrated computer-videotape recorder system is available.

We have used all of the listed methods, and each produced acceptable results. We formerly preferred the second method because of the reduction in labor involved in preparing the same images for projection slides and publication prints. More recently, however, we have upgraded to a computer-generated system (pg 125). If images are recorded on X-ray or diagnostic imaging film using a multiformat camera, slides can be prepared by rephotographing the transilluminated images.

Videotaping

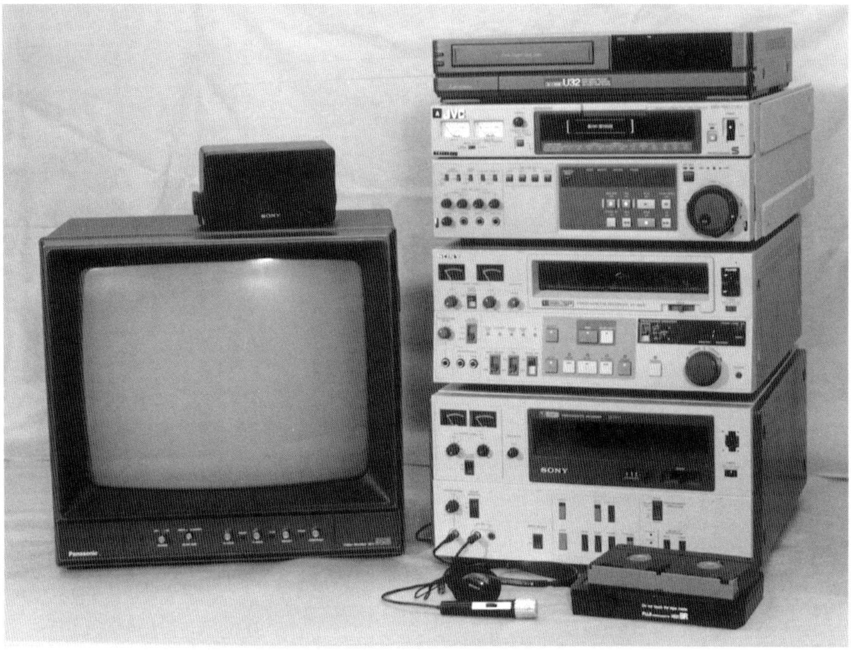

Videotape recorders and a video monitor. The four stacked videocassette recorders are as follows (top to bottom): conventional VHS half inch (Mitsubishi, HS-U32); Super VHS half inch (JVC Professional Products, BR-S622U); three-quarter inch (Sony, U-Matic SP, VO-9600); and three-quarter inch (Sony, U-Matic, VO-560). The monitor is a Panasonic Video Monitor, WV-5490.

Conventional VHS videocassette recorders use a one-half-inch format. They are inexpensive ($200 to $2,000, depending on options) and adequate for many purposes not requiring great detail. The resolution—approximately 230 lines of information—is less than for professional formats (discussed below). Most important, the system is widely used. A composite arrangement is used involving a combination of elements for color as well as black-and-white. Composite video is subject to signal degradation, which reduces image quality. Three-quarter-inch recorders have been used for research purposes because of higher resolution (at least 330 lines), time-code provisions, and image control (e.g., shuttle knob for low or high speed study and search capabilities). These recorders cost $4,000 to $7,000. However, since the methodology appears to be giving way to the Super-VHS format, good used machines and videotapes are becoming increasingly available at low cost. Thus, this format should be considered if high quality is a requirement but the budget is low.

Three-quarter-inch recorders have been the workhorse of the video industry for more than 20 years because of the high quality but apparently are being phased out.

Research laboratories that are upgrading appear to be favoring the Super-VHS format. This system uses special half-inch cassettes but also will play a conventional half-inch tape. The composite video arrangement of conventional half-inch recorders has been replaced by a format involving separation of the black-and-white and color functions, thereby reducing the signal degradation characteristic. The resolution of Super VHS is greater than 400 horizontal lines, compared with 300 lines for the three-quarter-inch format. The price range is $2,000 to $5,000 and involves many options. Portable, lightweight machines are available and are useful for recording at the scanning site. Super-VHS recorders are especially adaptable for editing and for frame-by-frame analyses. Broadcast-quality video systems use one- and two-inch digital videotape formats but are prohibitively expensive (e.g., $50,000) for routine taping of ultrasound images.

Videotape recording is an excellent means of storing real-time ultrasound scans. Video recorders may easily be connected to ultrasound instruments that have digital scan converters and video monitors. However, tape recorders cannot be used with older scanners that have analog scan converters (pg 61). Many ultrasound examinations can be stored on a single videotape. For example, 12 five-minute scans may be made on a one-hour three-quarter-inch tape. Half-inch videotapes in VHS format can store 2, 4, or 6 hours of examinations, depending upon the tape speed. However, there is a loss of image quality when extended-play recording options are used.

Taped ultrasound scans can be reviewed on the video monitor of the scanner or on a separate monitor. Household television sets are adequate for most purposes. However, if more detail is desired, high-resolution monitors are used. High-resolution monitors are loosely defined as having more than 500 lines. Most commercial high-resolution monitors have 650 to 850 lines of resolution. High-quality monitors generally have underscan capability, which allows all the information recorded on the videotape to be displayed on the monitor screen. When standard-scan monitors, such as a conventional television set, are used, there is a loss of 10 to 15 percent of the information at the periphery. In lower-quality monitors, imprecise registration of the projection system causes "blooming," or distortion of the image. Exceedingly high contrast settings also may result in blooming. The types of adapters for attaching scanners, monitors, and the various types of recorders can be confusing, and consultation from distributors of the products may be required.

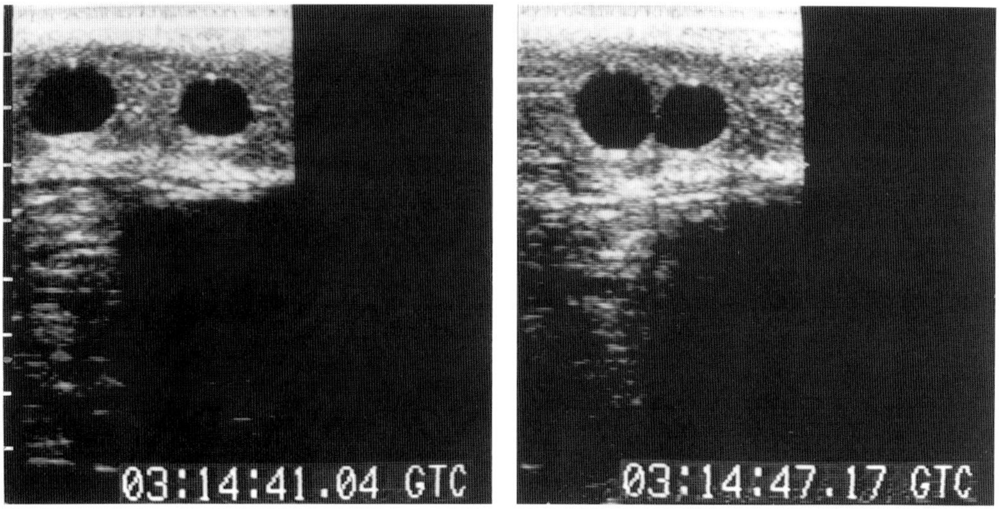

Sequential photographs from a videotape with time coding. The time code is placed on each frame, as shown. The numbers indicate (left to right) the tape number, minutes, seconds, and frame number (30 frames/second). Note that the two images that were selected for photography were taken at an interval of approximately 6.5 seconds. The time recordings show the overall movement of twin equine embryonic vesicles relative to one another during this time.

We routinely install time code on the video track of a duplicate videotape and in the audio track of the original tape. Thus, the original tape does not contain distracting numbers, but precise frames can be identified by reference to the coded copy. Also, time code can be inserted on channel 2 of the auditory system, thus leaving channel 1 available for on-site commentary. Time code is an eight-bit signal that is placed on the tape by a time-code generator and represents an industrial standard for elapsed time. The code is generated at 2,400 bits per second; 80 bits per frame at 30 frames per second (video play speed). There are even and odd fields for each frame. Time code is a highly accurate 24-hour clock that establishes precisely the time for each frame. An individual frame or series of frames can be located easily in the visual field with this system. Computerized editing facilities with the time code displayed on the videotape machine also can be used. The time-code system is very useful for editing or for analyzing motion, as in the assessment of uterine contractions or conceptus mobility.

Integration of a Scanner with a Computer

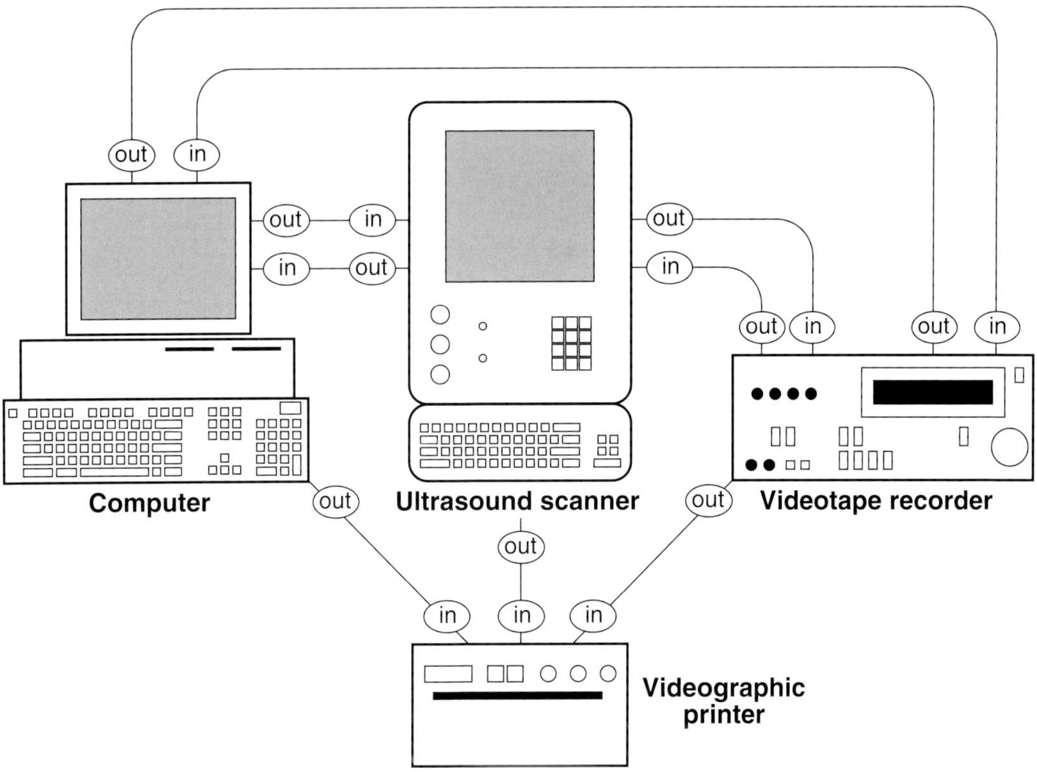

An example of integration. Ultrasonic scanners can be integrated with computers, tape recorders, and printers. Computer processing of ultrasonic image information continues to develop rapidly. A discussion on the use of computer software for obstetric sonography of the human fetus and the integration of computers and scanners is available and can be used as an introduction to this emerging area *(45)*. After the information (e.g., from videotapes) undergoes digitization, the data can be quantified, refined, or analyzed.

A system (Medimage) that will take images from a video source and store them in a personal computer is being marketed for animal work by Corometrics (source information: pg 191). The digitized images can be retrieved and processed. Examples of uses or processing include: 1) side-by-side or overlay comparisons; 2) transmittal by telephone; 3) enhancing, enlarging, filtering; 4) colorizing according to gray-scale; and 5) preparing projection slides for lectures or prints for publication. Other work stations and software systems for image processing are available *(12)*. Methods are described elsewhere for the use of digital image analyses of pixels for generating numerical data for assessing size and shape (e.g., follicles; pg 166) and echogenicity of gray scale (e.g., corpus luteum; pg 164).

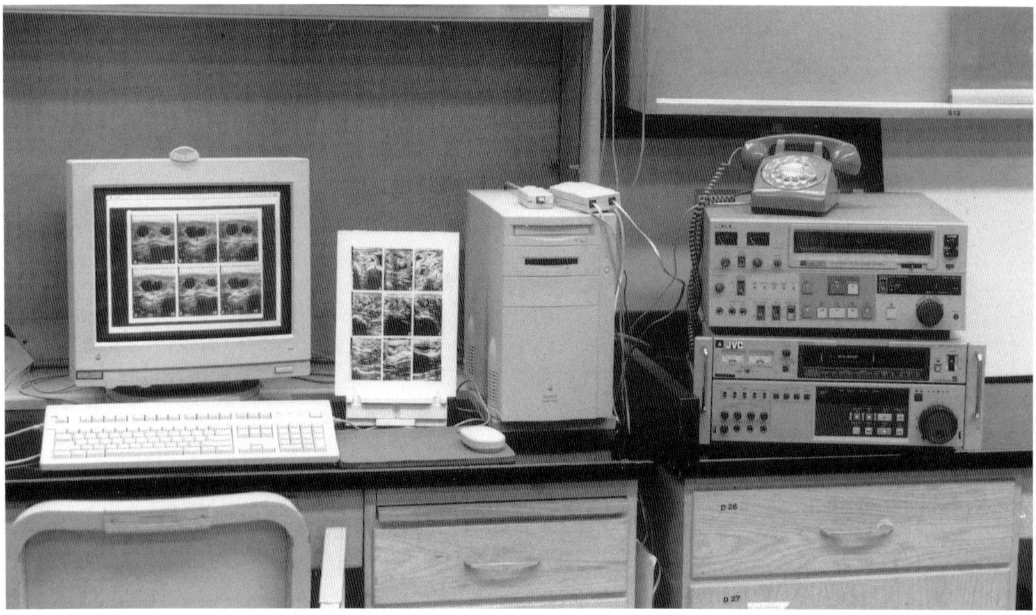

A computer-videotape workstation. The computer is a Quadra-840 AV by MacIntosh. Selected images can be processed and arranged, if desired, into panels for publication purposes using an Adobe Photoshop program. The panels then can be labeled with an Adobe Illustrator program. The electronic file then is sent to a digital processing laboratory for production of projection slides and photographic prints for publication. A discussion of techniques for preparing computer-generated slides was recently published in the Ultratalk Section of Veterinary Radiology and Ultrasound (Volume 35, Number 2, 1994). Examples of plates of multiple sonograms prepared with this station are shown elsewhere (pg 82, pg 102). Also, the result of processing the series of ultrasonograms depicted on the computer screen is shown (pg 26). Images processed through this system also can be displayed by a high-quality laser printer, especially for in-house purposes.

Apparently, three-dimensional imaging workstations are becoming available. They employ dedicated software to process and modify the digital data of two-dimensional images. Shading, shadowing, and smoothing are used to create the appearance of depth (see Veterinary Radiology and Ultrasound, Volume 34, Number 5, 1993).

Storage on Disks

An image stored in digital form can be transferred to disks *(106)*. Floppy disks are inexpensive and can store about 12 images. Hard disks can store a few hundred images. They may be offered as an integral component in a scanner for storing recent scans. As a guide, the number of images that can be stored on a disk is equivalent to capacity (megabytes) multiplied by four *(106)*; that is a 20 megabyte disk holds 80 images. Digital disks are not yet widely used in ultrasonic scanning.

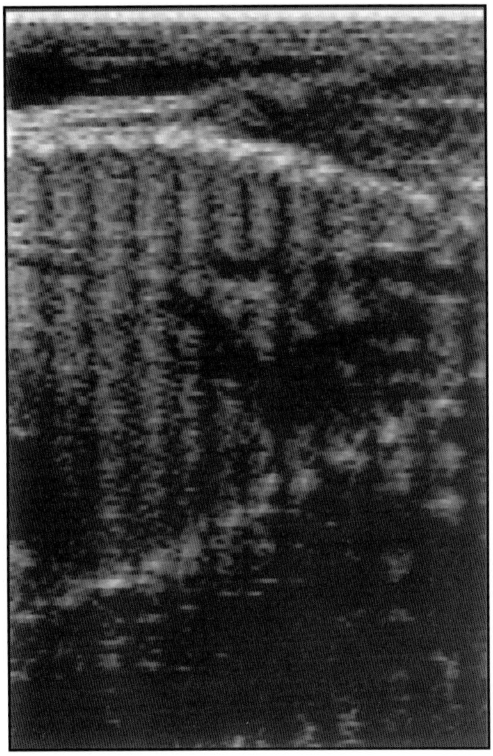

Imprisoned

Shadow artifacts from cross-sections of the fetal ribs in a 190-day equine fetus.

Chapter 8

TECHNIQUES

Attainment of the maximum capabilities of ultrasound instruments requires not only proper adjustments of the controls but also good scanning techniques. The operator must develop a thorough and realistic mental impression of the anatomy and orientation of the organs. Orientation is especially important in transrectal imaging of the uterus and ovaries because of organ mobility. The quality of transrectal imaging, like that of transrectal palpation, varies among examinations. Influencing factors include animal disposition and conformation, fat layers, intestinal gas pockets, and relationships among reproductive and other abdominal organs.

This chapter considers types of examining areas. Modern animal scanners are portable, but this technology nevertheless provides considerable incentive for the development of centralized work areas. Moving the scanner from animal to animal as in stanchion and tie barns is also considered. The purpose, preparation, and use of a coupling medium are discussed. Emphasis is given to transrectal examinations, but other approaches and techniques are noted, especially the rapidly expanding area of ultrasonic guiding of target-oriented instrumentation. The orientation of the organs for specific species and the effect on examining techniques will be reported in later texts of this series.

Transrectal Techniques

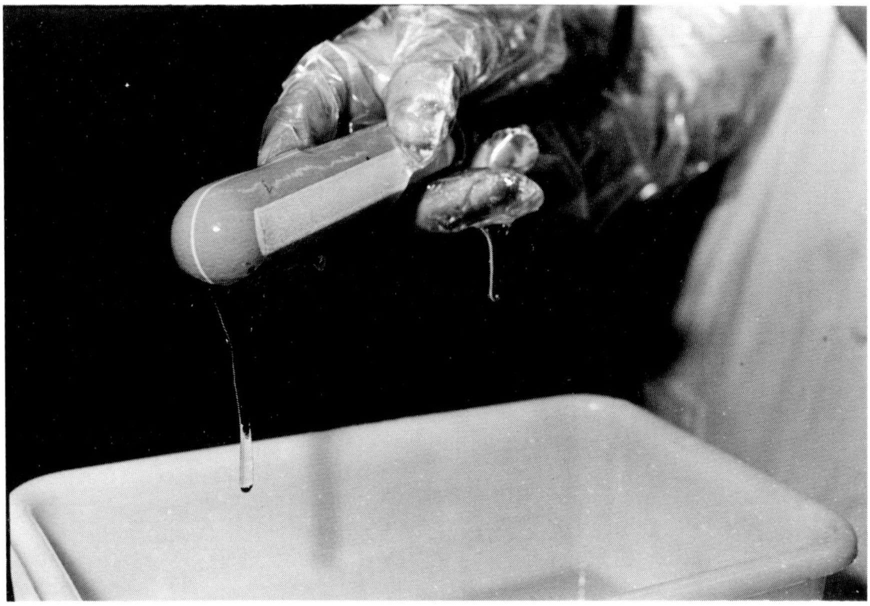

Dipping the transducer into coupling medium. The ultrasonic reflection coefficient of air approaches 100%. Therefore, air between the transducer face and the rectal wall blocks the entry of the ultrasonic pulses into the tissues *(pg 74)*. When a transducer is to be applied to skin, a hairless area is chosen (e.g., inguinal area) or the hair is clipped and a liberal application of a coupling medium is applied to prevent air interference. Because the rectal wall usually is moist, using a coupling medium is not as important for transrectal examinations. However, better contact sometimes is obtained if a coupling medium is used, especially when the animal's diet produces relatively dry fecal material. In addition, the coupling medium also serves as a lubricant, which is needed for intrarectal examinations. A water-soluble gel may be used for both lubricating and coupling. Certain substances, such as mineral oil or products containing an alcohol, should not be used because of potential transducer damage. The anal area is lubricated with the gel before inserting the hand, and the transducer is dipped into the gel. A gel may be prepared from carboxy-methylcellulose powder (source information: pg 196). The powder is combined with water using a mixer (e.g., paint mixer). One pound of powder will yield approximately five gallons of gel. Fecal material and excess gel should be removed from the transducer before they dry.

Inserting the lubricated hand and transducer into the rectum requires the same precautions that are used during rectal palpation to minimize rectal tears and ruptures. Presumably, ultrasound examination has an advantage over rectal palpation in preventing ruptures because folds of the rectal wall are not grasped as in palpating. Special precautions should be taken to ensure that the transducer is advanced within the lumen of the rectum and not into a blind pocket. This can be done by placing fingers beyond the tip of the transducer during major forward movements. For small animals (miniature horses, sheep, goats, immature animals), a rigid rod can be fastened to the probe to replace the oversized hand and arm. Some distributors of scanners may provide attachable extensions. With the extension approach, a contact gel or water can be inserted into the rectum with a syringe. Another method is to attach a tube to the probe and insert the contact medium as needed.

Preparing an animal for transrectal ultrasound examination (restraint, evacuation of rectum) is similar to preparing for transrectal palpation. Fecal material can cause distortions on the ultrasound image and must be removed. A pronounced shadow extending from the upper edge of the image may be due to intervening fecal matter (pg 70). If a structure does not image clearly, the face of the transducer is likely obscured by fecal debris or extraneous tissues are present between the organ and the rectal wall. If the transducer is hand-held, as in cattle and horses, debris may be removed by running a finger over the face of the transducer without removing the transducer from the rectum, and intervening tissue can be corrected by transrectal manipulation.

Each operator should develop a systematic procedure, depending on the species and whether the examination is to focus on selected areas or the entire tract. One approach, for example, is to examine the entire uterus and then the ovaries. This modification allows the operator to concentrate on locating specific structures or changes in a given organ. Details for examining certain organs or structures are given in subsequent texts in this series. During the examination, the viewing screen is the center of visual attention. At the same time, the location and orientation of the transducer and the resulting field of view are considered. This sense of hand-eye coordination, which relates the image to the tissues, becomes well-developed with experience.

In imaging in humans, a widely accepted convention exists for the orientation of an image on the display screen or photographic record (e.g., for longitudinal views, feet of patient are to the right side of screen; *106*). No such standardization has been adopted for transrectal imaging of the reproductive system of animals. Ultrasonograms are being published, for example, with the cranial orientation of the animal toward the left or right and, worse, it is often not stated what the orientation was. In these texts, the head is toward the left on all sonograms involving transrectal longitudinal examinations. We usually have the scanner positioned obliquely to the right side of the animal's rump, so that the left arm may be inserted into the animal, leaving the right hand free for writing and for adjusting the scanner. The actual orientation of the animal and the image (head to left) is therefore the same for all animals. Until a standard is developed, it is most important that operators in the same laboratory or veterinary practice agree on a common system.

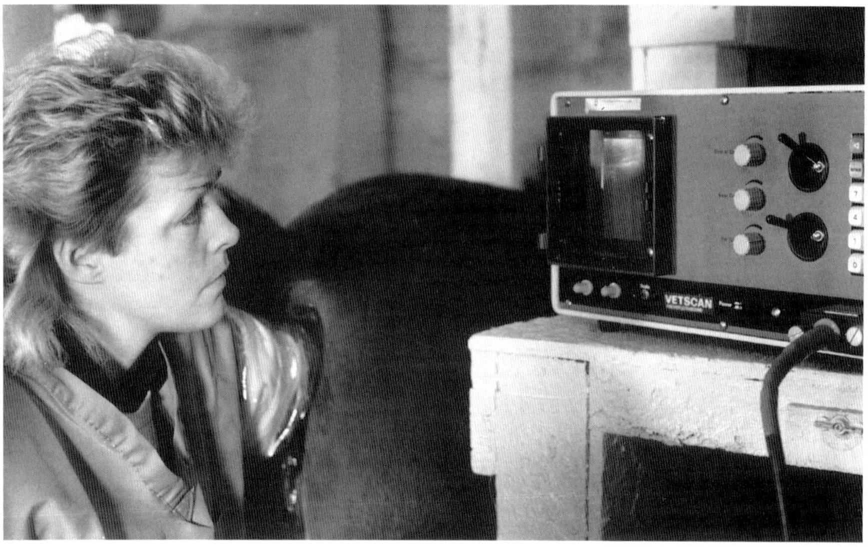

Close proximity of scanner to the sonographer's eyes. The height of the scanner's platform should position the scanner so that the screen and controls are approximately at eye level. The scanner should be close so that the controls can be adjusted and the details on the screen scrutinized by the operator while the transducer is being held in position. It is not uncommon to see published photographs with the operator in an uncomfortable position looking at a distant scanner setting, for example, on a hay bale. Simple procedures, such as equine pregnancy diagnosis after Day 15, probably can be accomplished in this manner. However, it is unlikely that the excitement and wonder of seeing an unusual detail will be experienced under such conditions. Occasionally, close scrutiny is diagnostically important (e.g., distinguishing a uterine cyst from an embryonic vesicle).

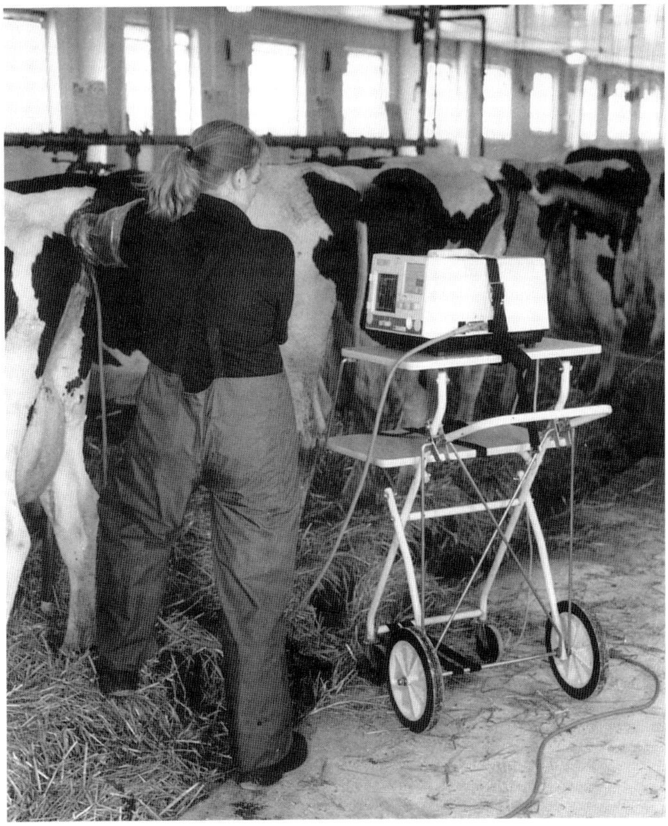

Scanning animals secured in rows or stalls. Dairy cattle are commonly held in stanchions or tie stalls. If an efficient centralized area is not available, the scanner can be moved from animal to animal. If properly designed, this approach can rival or exceed the efficiency of a centralized chute. Many distributors of portable scanners sell carts for this purpose (source information: pg 195). Some features of carts to consider are the following: 1) platform height that will bring the scanner screen closer to eye-level; 2) large, wide-based rear wheels so that the stand is stable and easy to move even over rough floors or ground; 3) good collapsibility for easy transportation or storage; 4) a second shelf for record books, towels, bucket, gloves, gel, etc; and 5) provisions for strapping the scanner to the cart. A professional cart is a small investment ($300 to $400) when measured against the value of the equipment that it holds and protects. A long extension cord (e.g., 15 meters) can be unrolled as the cart is moved. The cord of the scanner (not the extension cord) should be fastened to the cart so that the electric connection does not fall in water and so that the cord will disconnect if accidentally pulled. Conventional utility carts that are not designed for this purpose should not be used routinely, especially under barn conditions.

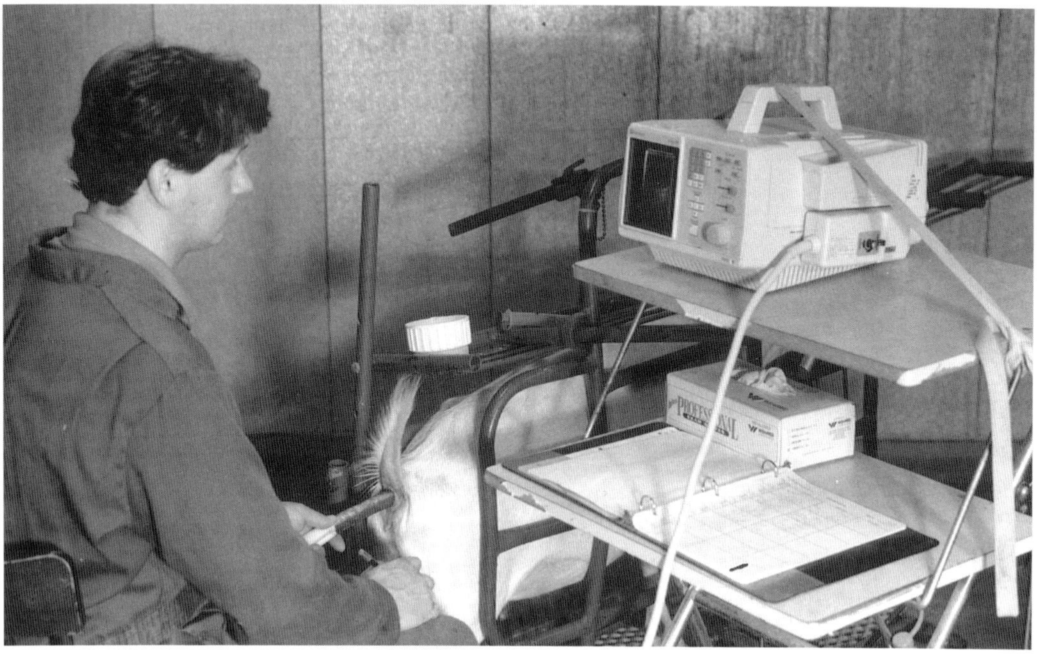

Examining stalls for small ruminants. Goats, sheep, and llamas can be led into an examining stall or cradle and the animals scanned while they are standing. In this example, the operator is seated behind the animal. A rigid rod has been fastened to the probe for external manipulation. A liberal quantity of contact gel can be inserted into the rectum before examination.

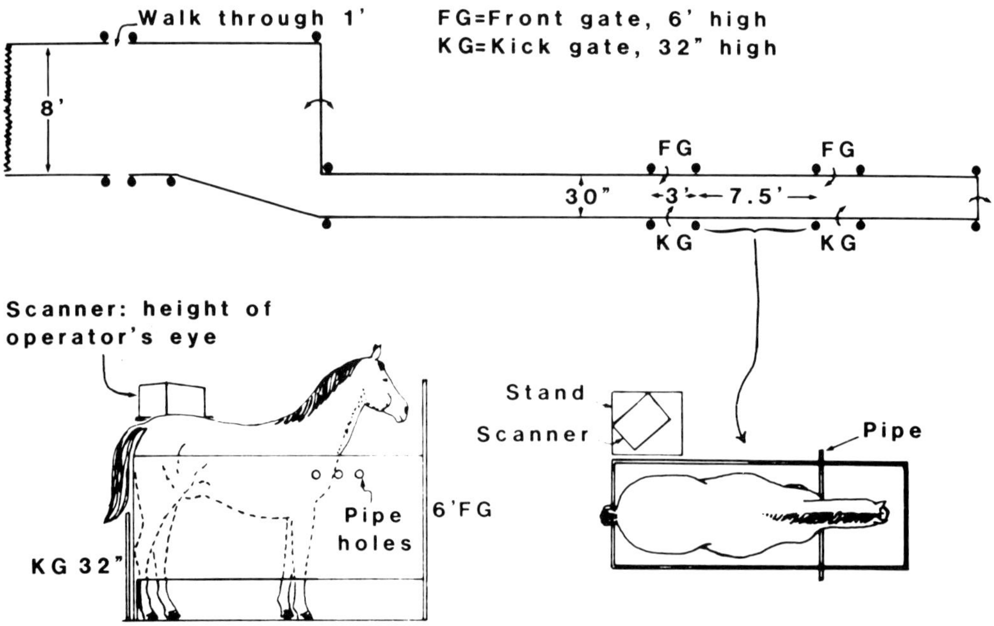

Centralized work area (facing page). Although modern veterinary ultrasound scanners are portable, they provide much incentive for the development of centralized examining areas. A centralized area will decrease the need for scanner transport and the dangers of damage—an important consideration. In this example, mares are corralled as a group in an area which leads into a long lane that terminates in one or more restraining chutes. If preferred, an individual mare can be led into an isolated chute.

A platform or cabinet can be built next to the rear of the chute, as shown. If the scanner is to stay with the farm, a cabinet can be built around the permanent scanner platform to enclose the scanner when not in use and thereby protecting it from damage and dust. When the scanner is in use, air must be able to circulate around it to prevent heat damage. The platform should be independent of the chute, so that it will not vibrate when the animal moves. Selection of the method of restraint and the design of an examining area must give consideration to the protection of the instrument as well as those who will use it. Subdued light is another requirement, and this will be well-known to anyone who has attempted to watch television outdoors. Image details are diminished or obliterated if the screen is directly exposed to light. Light from doors and windows should not hit the screen directly and should not hit the operator's eyes when the screen is being viewed. Working in an area that is too bright may encourage the operator to increase the gain to brighten the screen, thereby encouraging artifacts. Examination areas that were designed primarily for rectal palpation may therefore require some modifications.

The use of a separate electric circuit may help reduce interference from simultaneous use of electric appliances (e.g., refrigerators). The electric outlets at farm sites can be checked with a socket checker that can be purchased readily. These inexpensive devices will determine if the wiring was properly installed. If the wires were crossed during installation, the machine could be damaged. If the outlet is not grounded, the animal or operator can be shocked. The shocks can be imperceptible or barely perceptible to the operator, but disturbing to the animal. An electric surge protector should be an integral part of the scanner's electric plug.

Water Bath and Standoff Techniques

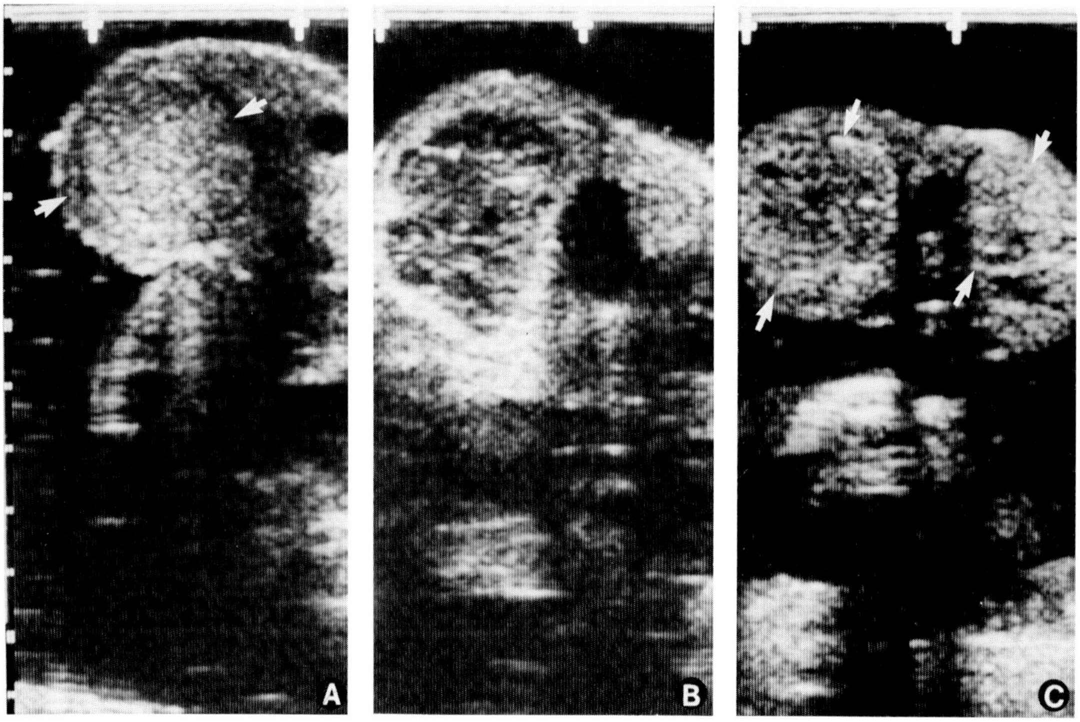

Images of excised equine ovaries taken in a water bath. A) Mature, solid corpus luteum (arrows); B) Corpus hemorrhagicum filled with a blood clot and fibrinous network; C) Two solid corpora lutea (arrows). The images were taken with the transducer applied to excised ovaries in a water bath. The ovaries were manipulated by grasping the mesovarium so that the fingers did not obscure the areas of interest. Artifacts are more of a problem in water baths because of reflective surfaces, especially when the imaging field encounters the sides of the container or air bubbles from recent agitation. The water-bath technique is especially useful for research and education. The water serves as a coupling medium, excluding air between the transducer face and the surface of the ovaries. Because water is an excellent conductor of electricity, manufacturers should be consulted regarding the insulating properties of their transducers. Cracked transducers or those with faulty insulation between the transducer and connecting cable should not be used. For educational purposes or to study the echotexture of certain structures, the tissue can be sliced in a plane approximating that of an image. Research uses include counting and classifying ovarian follicles without destroying the ovaries, and locating certain structures within organs as an aid in sampling for assay (e.g., follicular fluid) or histologic purposes. Tissues that have been fixed for histology can be examined by moving the tissue to a container of physiological saline (pg 103). We use this technique to locate embryos within a fixed uterus as an aid to histologic sectioning. In addition to direct scanning in a water bath, the probe can be applied with the aid of a contact gel to the exterior surface of a fluid-filled plastic container.

The standoff technique can be used when the transducer face is too close to the area of needed tissue information *(16)*. Because of the length of the ultrasonic pulse, there is a dead space of a few millimeters immediately next to the transducer face (e.g., 2 to 5 mm for a 3MHz probe). The dead space will encompass the rectal wall in transrectal imaging and because of close proximity may also obscure the surface or outer limits of the uterus or ovaries. If it is necessary to correct this problem (e.g., a specialized research need), a layer of water or gel can be trapped around the probe in a hollow tube or thin rubber sheath *(106)*. Alternatively, a commercially available standoff material can be mounted on or held beneath the transducer face. The standoff technique also can be used for examining excised tissues.

Other Techniques

We are entering a galaxy of ultrasound technologies in human medicine. These techniques are briefly noted here because, presumably, they could be adapted and creatively used for research and clinical evaluations in animal reproduction.

Endoluminal transducers or ultrasonic endoscopes are used to inspect the internal lining or adjacent tissues of tubular organs *(106)*. In reality, transrectal ultrasonic viewing of the reproductive tract of large animals is a form of this technique; bone, muscle, and fat are bypassed, and the transducer is placed close to the organ of interest. Both linear-array and rotating transducers have been built into the end of optical video-endoscopic tubes. The inside wall of the organ can be viewed optically, and structures beneath the surface or adjacent to the tubular organ can be viewed ultrasonically. For example, the human pancreas can be imaged through the stomach wall. Presumable, such a device could be used to inspect the internal surface of the equine uterus as well as the deeper wall (e.g., cysts, endometrial cups). The uterus could be filled with water or a water-filled balloon on the tip of the probe could be used to provide acoustic coupling. A balloon in available models moves the closest scanned structures 1 or 2 cm from the transducer face; focusing is improved and reverberations are minimized.

A variety of miniature ultrasound transducers has been developed for endoluminal use *(82)*. The transducers are placed in catheters of a few millimeters in diameter and inserted into the lumens of vascular and nonvascular structures. The instruments have frequencies of 12.5 to 20 MHz and are used to locate smaller intraluminal abnormalities. In the past few years, they have been used in humans to inspect the lining of blood vessels, urethra, urinary bladder, esophagus, and oviducts. Recent advances in computer technology have raised the capability of using endoluminal ultrasound for producing 360° cross-sectional images at set intervals resulting in multiple planes. The multiple images can be digitally stored and computer-reconstructed to produce a three-dimensional image (pg 126). We are not aware of the use of miniature endoluminal transducers in large-animal theriogenology, but researchers, especially, should be aware of this recent innovation.

Intraoperative sonography is becoming increasingly popular in the human field, and small linear array transducers designed specifically for such use are available *(104)*. The technique is used to further evaluate and delineate abnormal areas that cannot be studied adequately by the exterior route. Presumably, the linear array transducers, especially those of 5.0 or 7.5 MHz, designed for intrarectal placement in large animals would be suitable for this purpose. Gas sterilization of the transducer and coaxial cable is recommended; 12 to 36 hours are required. As an alternative, a sterile plastic or latex sleeve can be used. Covers that fit specific transducers are available. When ultrasonic scanning is to be done after a laparotomy, effort should be made to remove air from the abdomen in conjunction with suturing the incision *(130)*.

Transabdominal Technique

Although this series of books is devoted primarily to transrectal examination of the reproductive tract, the transabdominal approach is an option that should not be overlooked and is the primary approach for small animals. The Doppler principle (pg 23, pg 109) has been used for transabdominal and transrectal detection of fetal or uterine blood flow in animals, but results have been limited *(reviews: 144, 169)*. Transabdominal A-mode scanning (pg 23) provides an indication of the depth of interfaces beneath the skin surface. The A-mode has been used as a pregnancy indicator but has given limited and variable results. Real-time, B-mode pregnancy scanning by the transabdominal route, using a linear array transducer, was reported in dogs in 1983 *(20)* and in sheep in 1984 *(173)* and has been extended to cats *(43)*, goats *(review: 100)*, and llamas *(115)*. Sheep may be held in a dorsal or sitting position, and the probe is moved across the width of the abdomen approximately 20 cm in front of the udder; some operators clip the wool in the area *(144)*. Sector scanning is also used for this purpose, usually with the animal standing. Pregnancy can be diagnosed on the basis of a fluid-filled uterus at 30 days and fetuses can be detected at 45 to 50 days *(144)*. Goats and llamas are handled in the standing position.

In pigs, reports on real-time transabdominal pregnancy diagnosis began to appear in the literature in 1983 *(review: 157)*. Apparently, linear array transducers are preferred because the pregnant uterus is close to the transducer; most reports involved a 3.5 or 5.0 MHz transducer. The probe is placed on the ventral abdominal wall just above the row of teats and immediately cranial to the hindlimb *(21)*. The fluid-filled uterus can be detected at 20 to 30 days as anechoic areas *(157)*.

The transabdominal route is used for pregnancy diagnosis and evaluation of the internal reproductive system in dogs and cats *(reviews: 158, 177)*. The transducer is placed midventrally between the rows of teats. First examinations for pregnancy are often done 26 to 30 days after the first mating.

A transabdominal approach can be used to image the equine fetus after 100 days *(114, 132)*. In the most extensive study *(132)*, excessive hair was clipped and a coupling gel was used. The transducers (2.5 to 3.0 MHz) were placed in the inguinal area. Fetal parts, amniotic fluid, placental membranes, and motion patterns were imaged. Fetal heart rates decreased from 180 beats/minute at 100 days to 60 to 80 beats/minute two weeks before parturition. It was concluded that this approach was practical in later pregnancy for detecting fetal orientation and viability and the presence of twins. The transabdominal approach has been used to eliminate one member of a fetal-twin set by ultrasonically guided injections into the fetal heart. We were unable to image the fetus with this approach in fat ponies using a 3.5 MHz transducer. Perhaps the known deleterious effects of fat on ultrasonic beams interferes with the practicality of this approach in fat mares.

Simulated Structures, Markers, and Contrast Media

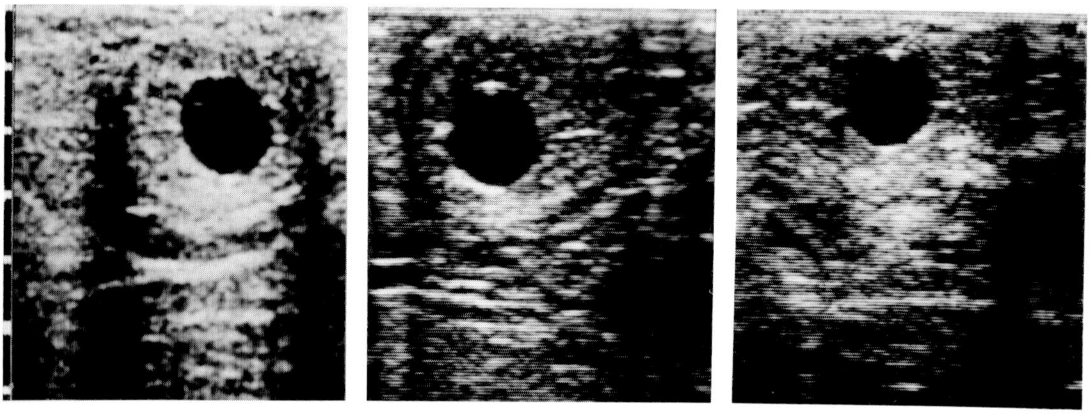

Simulated structures. Simulated embryonic vesicles are being used to study the mechanisms involved in intrauterine mobility of the equine embryo *(56)*. The vesicles are made by injecting water into small rubber balloons made from the fingertips of surgical gloves. The figure shows a Day-13 equine embryonic vesicle (left) and a simulated vesicle in a uterine horn (middle) and 20 minutes later in the uterine body (right). This approach was used to show that even inanimate objects are mobile in the uterus but the rate of movement was not as rapid as for embryonic vesicles.

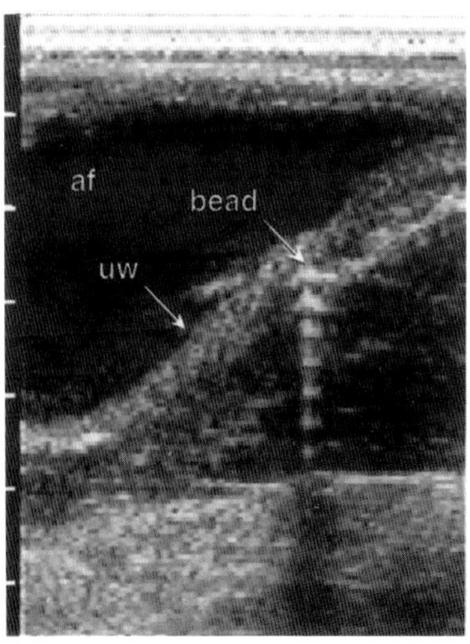

Echogenic markers. af=allantoic fluid. uw=uterine wall (internal surface). Echogenic objects (e.g., 5 mm steel beads) can be placed or sutured to a given location for experimental ultrasonic monitoring of a specific area. The sonogram shows the reverberations beneath the image of a 5 mm steel bead that was sutured to the external wall on the ventral aspect of an equine, gravid uterine body. The technique was used for monitoring the sequential transient changes in the height of the allantoic fluid *(84)*, thereby allowing in situ characterizations of allantoic fluid shifts.

Contrast media are being used to highlight lumens, cavities, or vessels for ultrasonic imaging in humans. At present, this approach is primarily experimental. Microbubbles are produced when a watery solution is agitated. These air-filled bubbles are readily imaged and serve to confirm the location of injection needles and catheters during interventional procedures (pg 143). Because of the bubble and scatter (pg 33) phenomena, we have been able to observe the arrival of semen into the uterus through an infusion pipette or an experimental solution into a follicle through a small (25 gauge) transvaginal needle. Free gas bubbles are excellent scatterers of an ultrasound beam because of the pronounced mismatch between gas and tissue. Gas bubbles occur during agitation of a fluid and are a common nuisance in water bath studies, especially immediately after preparation of the bath. Free-gas bubbles have the disadvantage of being short-lived. Uniform, small gas bubbles also have been produced by a procedure known as sonification *(143)*.

A commercial product called SHU 454 is being used as an ultrasonic contrast agent *(88)*. This agent is a powdered polysaccharide that forms a microbubble suspension when mixed with a diluent. It has been used intravenously; the carrier sugar is metabolized by the liver. It also has been used for highlighting lumens and cavities. Notable among these is a system for testing patency of the oviducts by transvaginal ultrasound-guided injections into the uterus *(44, 88)*. This technique is said to be a simple screening method for tubal patency in women, and perhaps should be investigated as a possible technique in farm species. Several other contrast agents also offer promise for improved ultrasonic diagnostic accuracy and as a research aid. These include gelatin encapsulated nitrogen microspheres, indocyamine green, Albunex (commercial microbubble preparation of serum albumen), colloidal suspensions (solid particles suspended in a liquid), and lipid emulsions; those interested in these products can consult recent reviews (e.g., *88*). In addition to highlighting and testing patency of the oviducts, another potential use of a contrast agent in animals is to mark a specific ovarian follicle that has been given an experimental preparation.

Ultrasonic Guiding

Instrument	Target	Payload	Examples of uses
1. Needle			
A. Aspiration	Follicle	Oocytes Follicular fluid Granulosa	IVF, anatomical studies Hormonal assessment Tissue culture, hormonal and anatomical assessment
	Fetal heart or blood vessels	Blood	Genetic evaluation, biochemical and serological studies
	Maternal vessels	Blood	Hormonal studies of specific organs
	Pathological structures	Fluid	Differential diagnosis
	Allantois	Fluid	Physiological studies
	Amnion	Fluid with cells	Genetic evaluation, physiological studies
	Uterus	Fluid	Physiological and pathological studies
	Yolk sac or allantois	Fluid	Twin reduction
B. Insertion	Follicles	Hormones, biochemicals oocytes	Physiological studies
	Uterus	Embryo Hormones, biochemicals Antibiotics, drugs	Transfer Physiological studies Therapy
	Conceptus (heart, fluids)	KOH or other fetocidal agent	Twin reduction
	Pathological areas	Antibiotics, drugs	Local therapy
2. Biopsy tool	Chorion	Villi	Genetic evaluation
	Any accessible tissue or area	Tissue sample	Anatomical, physiological and pathological studies
3. Cannula	Vessels, cavities, lumens	Indwelling cannula	Chronic sampling, delivery, or drainage
4. Cauterizing instrument	Any accessible area	---------------	Ablation or cauterization

Table of demonstrated and potential uses of ultrasonic guiding (facing page). Ultrasonic guiding is ideally suited for placing needles and other instruments within targets in the body because of the real-time aspects and safety. This has become the method of choice for puncture guidance in the human field. Computed tomography is also used but is usually reserved for targets obscured by bone *(92)*. Real-time needle guidance systems have been used in humans since the late 1970s. In large-animal theriogenology, the use of scanners to position a biopsy instrument in the equine uterus was reported in 1986 *(58)*, and the potential for guiding needles into various structures in animals was extolled. The results of a needle-guiding study were not reported, however, until 1988 *(131)*; this illustrates the long delay that commonly occurs in using available technologies. Creative animal scientists should consider the wide array of ultrasound-guided techniques emerging in human medicine *(92)*. In large animals, linear-array *(26)*, convex array *(23, 36)*, and sector transducers have been adapted with needle guides for transvaginal aspiration of follicular fluid for the collection of oocytes. Initially, the purchase of a special transducer was required, but more recently, needle-guide assemblies became available for easy attachment. In using transvaginal probes, it should be noted that many coupling gels have been shown to be spermicidal *(149)*.

Ultrasonically guided biopsy has been used to obtain a localized biopsy within the equine uterus, using transrectal imaging as a guide *(58)*. However, more refined instrumentation is being used in humans and could be adapted for use in animals. Two types of biopsy instruments have been developed—fine-needle aspiration and large-needle core sampling *(89, 92, 120, 140)*. For the fine-needle technique, a 22-gauge needle can be used for obtaining cells for cytological work without risk of hemorrhage. Larger cores can be obtained with specially designed 14- or 18-gauge needles. Large-bore needles may be designed to cut either from the end or side of the needle. Side-cutting needles can be obtained that are used with an automated spring-loaded biopsy gun *(140)*. The resulting core sample can be prepared for histologic study of the tissue architecture. A modified system involves the replacement of the removed core with a plug to minimize hemorrhage. With large needles, the selection of a safe pathway is especially important.

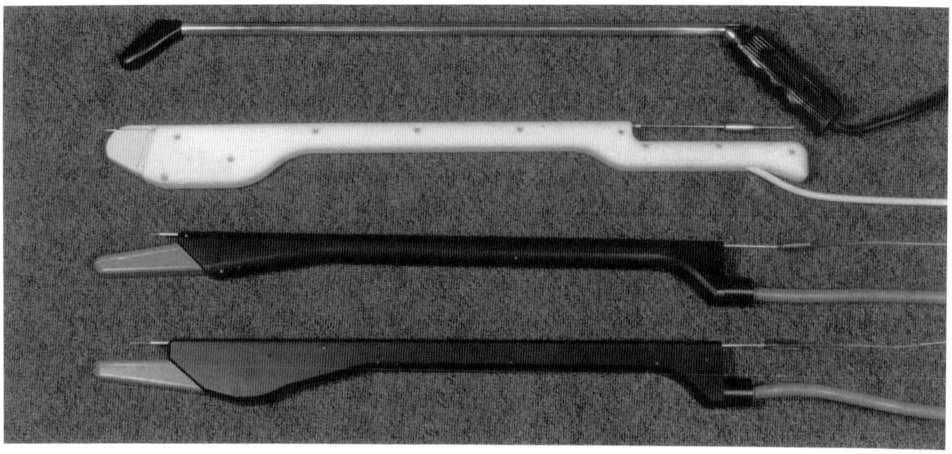

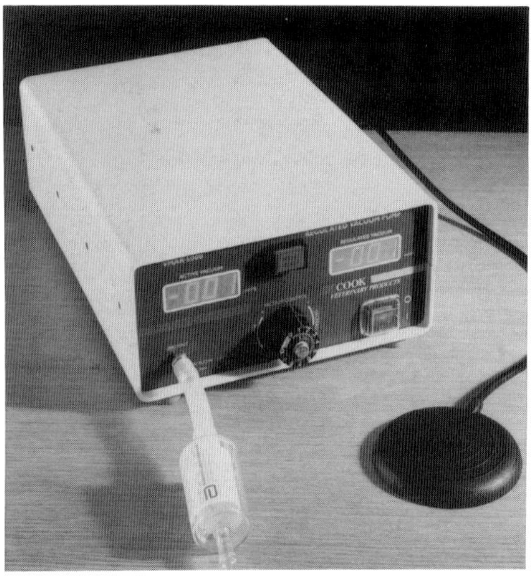

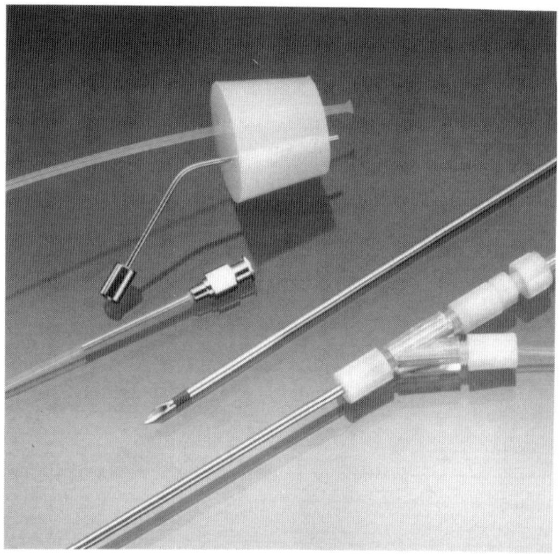

Paraphernalia for transvaginal ultrasonic guiding. Transvaginal aspiration of cattle and horse follicular oocytes for in vitro fertilization is becoming commonplace. Specialized convex and sector transducers and devices for encasing conventional linear-array transducers are being marketed (top to bottom: Pie Medical, Aloka, Tokyo Keiki, Tokyo Keiki; source information: pg 191). An aspiration pump and needles with adapters are also shown (Cook; source information: pg 195). Note the ultrasound etch mark near the needle's point. Increasing the reflectivity of the needle may be done by roughening the surface to increase the number of acoustic interfaces or by incorporating an air-containing notch near the needle tip. Such needles can be purchased, or a needle tip can be scarified with a fine file *(8)*. Another approach involves a simulated needle path on the ultrasound screen. Linear-array transducers or transducers that produce a longitudinal field of view display a clear image of the longitudinal aspects of the needle *(26)*: needles as small as 25 gauge were imaged within the follicular fluid.

Part Three

RESEARCH

Chapter 9

RESEARCH ASPECTS

In the short time that transrectal ultrasonic imaging of the reproductive tract has been used as a research tool, many discoveries have resulted, some of which would otherwise have escaped detection for many years (listing on pg 20). Before the introduction of real-time transrectal ultrasonic imaging in large-animal reproductive research, the morphology of the reproductive organs was evaluated by transrectal palpation, at surgery, or after excision. The dynamic aspects of morphology were largely inaccessible. Real-time ultrasonic imaging has provided a noninvasive and nondisruptive technique to image directly the changing internal and external anatomy of reproductive organs and tissues and to characterize reproductive events (e.g., ovulation, transition of the uterus from a diestrous to an estrous echotexture). A dynamic event (e.g., ovulation) can be monitored in entirety by continuous observation (e.g., 30 minutes), or examinations can be done repeatedly over many days. For example, recently we monitored growth and regression of individual follicles in goats, as described *(77)*, every day for one year, with no recognizable untoward side effects. Including ultrasonic examinations in experimental protocols provides the opportunity to associate changing morphology with hormonal and other functional changes. If experimental testing is expected to involve changing morphology—and it usually does—ultrasonic imaging should be considered. End points can be measured or ranked, and therefore data can be statistically analyzed for conventional hypothesis-testing. A review of statistical methods, as applied to ultrasonic end points, is available *(97)*. Clearly, the research potential of this technology and its adaptability for computer-assisted assessment go far beyond simplistic determination of ovulation, luteal formation, and pregnancy diagnosis.

Maximal use of ultrasonography requires good equipment and examining conditions, keen observational skills, and creative utilization. The techniques of simulating structures, marking specific areas (pg 140), and guiding insertion devices (e.g., insemination pipettes, biopsy or aspiration needles, pg 142) illustrate how the power of ultrasonography can be extended even further. Furthermore, the technology adds a measure of excitement to research because of the ability to observe dynamic reproductive events as they occur—including events that were previously unknown.

Ultrasonic Reference and End Points

Advantages of ovulation versus estrus as a reference point:

1. Readily and objectively detected
2. Encompasses a narrow time span
3. Represents a profound and central endocrinologic event
4. Detection requires little additional time, if the study involves ultrasonic examinations for other reasons

Ovulation as an ultrasonic reference point. Farm-animal biologists have traditionally used estrus as a primary reference point. Paradoxically, many researchers, even though they determine the day of ovulation ultrasonically, continue to report, for example, profiles of changing hormonal concentrations and follicular development using estrus as the reference or starting point. Behavioral criteria, as used for defining estrus, are difficult to standardize among and within laboratories, experiments, and investigators, whereas ultrasonically determined ovulation is objective. Moreover, ovulation can be confirmed by the development of a corpus luteum. The time of ovulation, in contrast to varying estrous lengths among animals and species, can be narrowly defined by ultrasound, limited only by the frequency of examinations. Furthermore, consideration can be given to multiple ovulations occurring at different times. Another advantage of ovulation as a reference point involves its partitioning of markedly different hormonal environments. The time required for determination of ovulation is minimal if efficient facilities are available (pgs 132 to 135). A program can be developed to decrease the need for daily examinations. For example, in mares, daily examinations need not begin until a follicle has reached 25 mm. If behavioral checks are replaced by ultrasonic monitoring for ovulation, the true length of the estrous cycle will be unknown. The length of the interovulatory interval can be used instead.

Other ovarian reference and end points that have become available solely through ultrasonography include the following: 1) day of emergence of a follicular wave, 2) day of divergence of follicles into dominant and subordinate categories, 3) beginning of regression of an anovulatory dominant follicle, and 4) beginning of morphologic luteolysis. Each of these characteristics will require a firm definition as part of the experimental protocol.

A reproductive reference and end point that was unimaginable in small and large-animal research before the introduction of ultrasonography is the establishment of the time of embryonic death. The embryonal heartbeat is obvious by Day 24, and detecting its cessation provides the scientist with one of the criteria used for death in adults. The precision is limited only by the frequency of examinations. It has not been determined whether altered embryonal or fetal heart rate can be detected prior to death as an indicator of stress or impending disaster. The heart rate does increase considerably during bouts of fetal activity in the equine fetus (unpublished observations).

In addition to the above discrete end points, many quantitative end points have become available through the imaging technology. Included are the following: 1) diameter, area, or growth and regression rates of follicles; 2) diameter or growth rate of the embryonic vesicle, embryo proper, and other measurable structures involving the conceptus; 3) diameter, area, or growth and regression rates of the corpus luteum; 4) heart rate; 5) rate of mobility of the embryonic vesicle in mares; 6) diameter or other measures of the uterus; and 7) height or other measures of fluid pockets in the uterus, vagina, and conceptus.

One of the delightful aspects of the ultrasound research technology is that it challenges and stimulates scientists to develop reference and end points for a specific study area—end points that have not been considered previously because no methodology existed for their assessment. Most research laboratories have not been reporting on statistical analyses, with probabilities, for ultrasonically derived data. This section and subsequent sections will demonstrate, however, that ultrasonic data can be handled similarly to data from other experimental data-gathering technologies. The primary difference is that ultrasound provides more choices than other technologies in the kinds of data that can be collected.

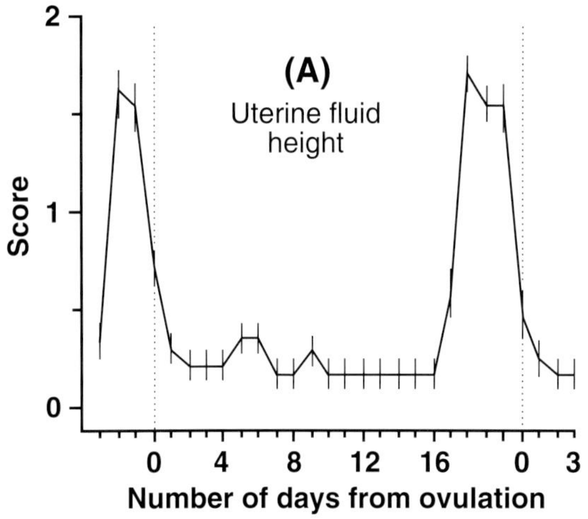

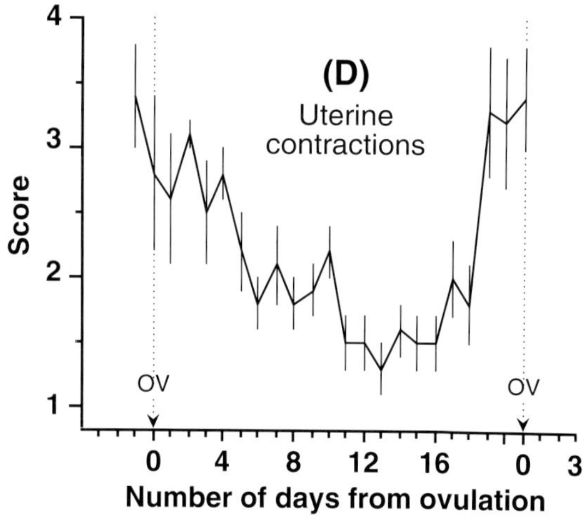

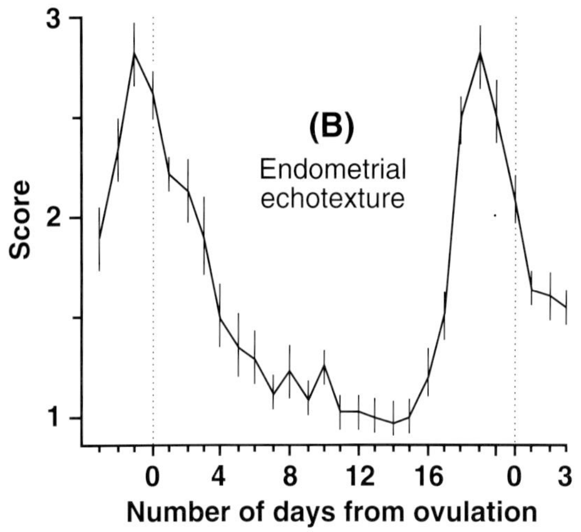

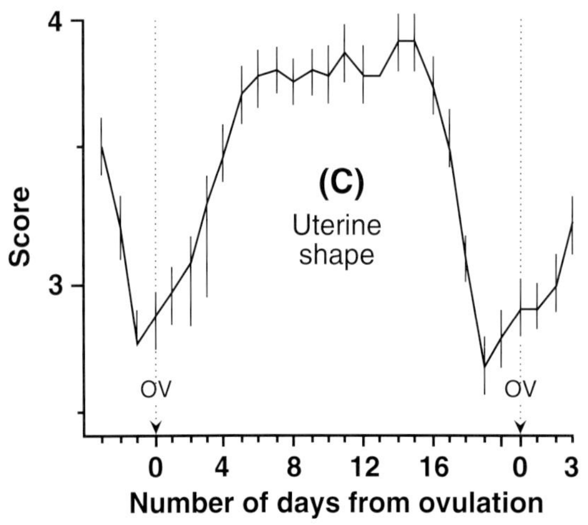

Scored end points.

(A) Relative quantity of accumulated intrauterine fluid (1=minimal, 2=intermediate, 3=maximal).

(B) Extent of endometrial edema as indicated by echotexture (1=minimal as seen during diestrus, 2=intermediate, 3=maximal as seen during estrus).

(C) Shape of the uterus or degree of spiraling (1=minimal, 2 and 3=intermediate, 4=maximal).

(D) Extent of uterine contractility (1=minimal, 2 and 3=intermediate, 4=maximal).

Many ultrasonic characteristics are not amenable conveniently to quantitation by conventional techniques. An approach that we have used extensively is to score the extent of a given event from minimal to maximal. The scored end points shown in the four figures are from studies in cattle *(19, 128)*. There was a significant day effect for each end point.

The scoring approach facilitates profiling and statistically analyzing changes during a time period (e.g., interovulatory interval) and analyzing the temporal relationships or correlations among the ultrasonically monitored events as well as among other events. Without a scoring system, the end points might not be accessible for statistical handling. The scoring system is subjective in that the sonographer's judgment is used. Subjectivity can be converted to objectivity, if deemed appropriate, by videotaping the images so that scoring can be done without knowledge of source, or scoring can be done by a second operator who is unaware of source or even the hypothesis under test.

We have developed considerable confidence in the scoring approach because of consistent results among experiments and independent operators and the ease of interpretation of results in relationship to known biological mechanisms. For example, a small, transient, significant surge in endometrial echotexture was detected in mares on Day 5 *(87)*; six years later, another laboratory found a secondary surge in urinary estrogens at this time *(42)*. We have consulted with statisticians who expressed concern that these discrete (discontinuous) end points were being analyzed by conventional analyses of variance, but other statisticians seemed less concerned. Most notably, we have used this approach for approximately 14 ultrasonically derived end points in cattle and horses in more than 40 publications and do not believe that we have been misled in any of our experimental results. That is, it has worked for us. Apparently, however, a method called categorical-data analysis or log-linear modeling has been developed in recent years. Although we have not yet used this method, it seems especially appropriate for ultrasonically derived scoring systems and should be considered. An advantage is that it provides an interaction term, similar to the results of factorial analyses of variance.

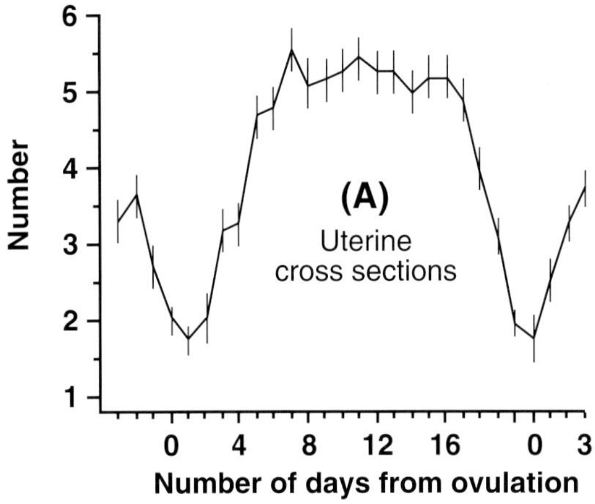

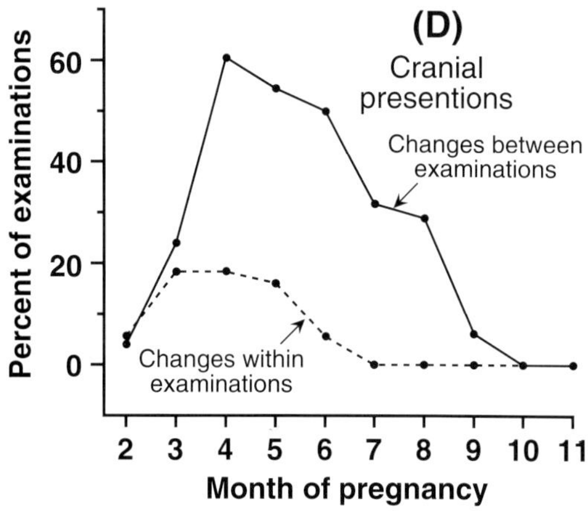

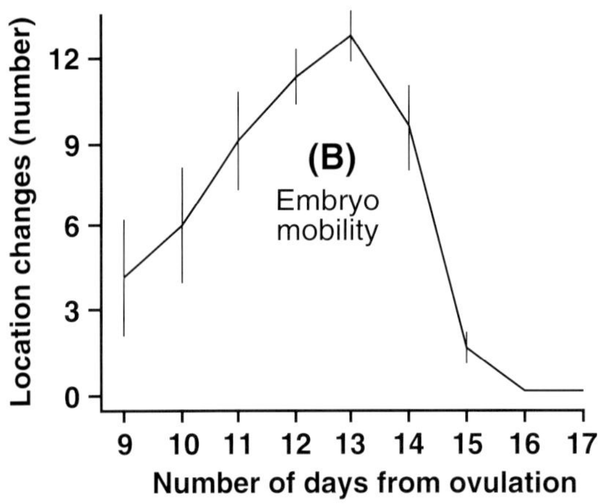

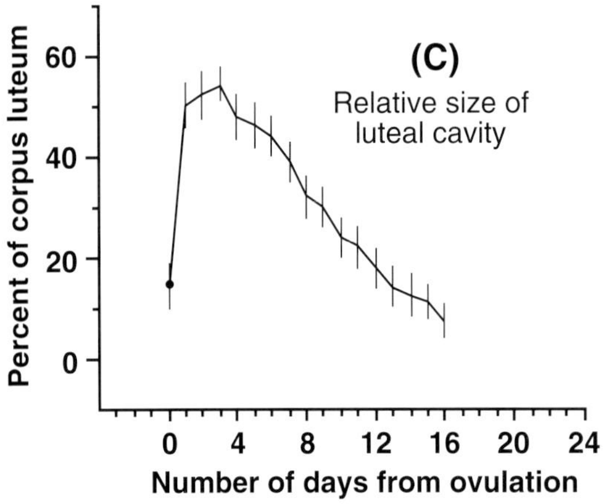

Ultrasonically derived end points involving number or frequency .

(A) Number of cross-sections of uterine horn in an ultrasonic field using a constant number of interovulatory intervals (n=58) per day in cattle. This end point was used as an expression of the changes in the degree of spiraling of the uterine horns during an interovulatory interval *(128)*.

(B) Mean number of times the equine embryonic vesicle changed locations over two hours on various days of early pregnancy *(101)*. Data are from two-hour trials in which location was determined every five minutes in each mare on each day. The uterine segments were the body and three approximately equal portions of each horn. In addition to number of changes from segment to segment, the number of changes from horn to horn or between horn and body were also used. Approaches involving number of changes per unit of time allow characterization of changes over days (e.g., changes in the extent of embryo mobility).

(C) Percentage of a luteal gland that consisted of an anechoic central area (blood clot) for various days in 26 interovulatory intervals in mares *(124)*. This analysis characterized the changing morphology of the corpus luteum.

(D) A depiction of the frequency of changes in fetal presentation in horses *(73)*. A five-minute ultrasonic examination was made every 3 or 4 days from Month 2 to parturition. The graph shows the frequency of presentation changes within a five-minute examination and the frequency of presentation changes from one examination to the next.

End points involving changes in the number or frequency of certain events are useful for characterization or temporality studies and for testing hypotheses. The frequency can be expressed conveniently in numbers of events when the total number is constant over time or as percentages when the numbers change. The figures illustrate the amenability of ultrasonic frequency data to statistical evaluation. The data for figures A, B, and C were analyzed by analyses of variance, using arc-sign transformation for the percentage data (C). The data for part D were analyzed for differences among months by chi-square analyses, using the numbers from which the percentage for each month was derived.

Centralization and Normalization

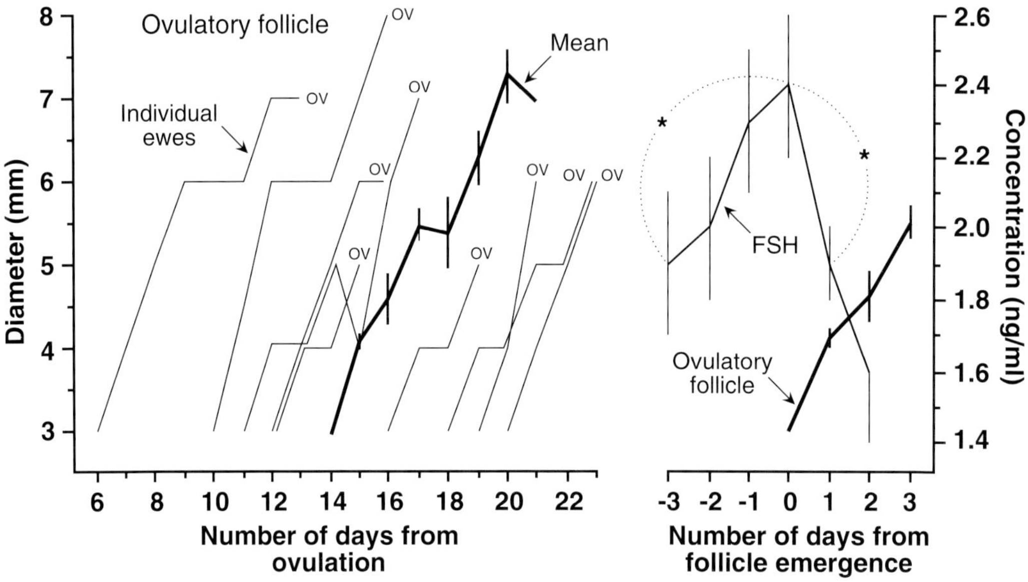

Growth profiles for ovulatory follicles. OV=ovulation. The follicle diameters for nine individual ewes are shown on the left panel, extending from follicle emergence at 3 mm to ovulation. The observations were taken from the raw data of a reported study *(76)*. The follicles emerged at different times, and the mechanisms associated with emergence would be difficult to assess unless all follicles were assigned to a common day of emergence. This can be done by <u>centralization</u>, using the mean day of emergence (heavy line). To study the temporal relationship of another event (changes in FSH concentrations) to the emergence of the follicles, the FSH values were carried with the corresponding follicle values for each ewe, so that the values for both end points were associated with the mean day of follicle emergence. In this manner, it was demonstrated that, on the average, a significant (starred dotted line between two means) increase in FSH concentrations preceded the emergence or growth of follicles from 3 to 4 mm. <u>Normalization</u> can be used to standardize the length of the interovulatory interval, for example. The mean length of the interval is used for the day axis; days are randomly deleted or added (using missing values) to each individual's data so that they conform to the normalized day scale. Although these statistical maneuvers are used commonly with other characteristics (e.g., hormone values), few laboratories, according to literature reports, apply them to values derived by ultrasonic imaging. It is important to recognize that data from ultrasonic imaging can be processed and analyzed like data from other instrumentation.

Temporality

P = Peak FSH value
E = Emergence of ovulatory follicle

Ewe	Relative FSH values/day	No. days P to P	No. days from E to nearest P: Observe	No. days from E to nearest P: Expect
1	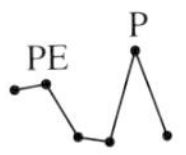	3	0	0.7
2	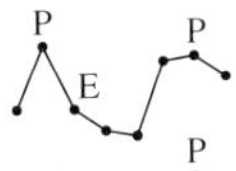	5	1	1.2
3	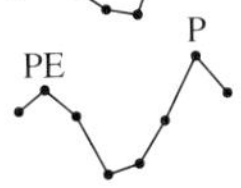	5	0	1.2
4	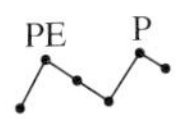	3	0	0.7
5	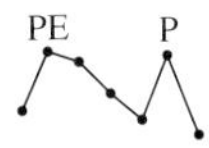	4	0	1.0
6	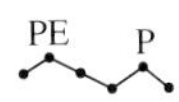	3	0	0.7
7	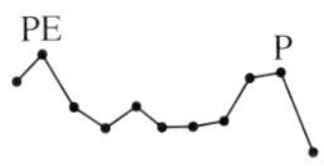	8	0	2.0
8	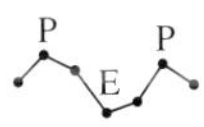	4	2	1.0
9	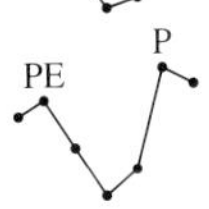	4	0	1.0
			0.3 ±0.2	1.1 ±0.1

Determining the probability that two events are temporally related. These data are from the study *(76)* considered on the facing page. The extent of temporality between day of emergence of the ovulatory follicle and the peak value of an FSH fluctuation involves the shortest distance (days) between the two events; the FSH peaks were detected by a cycle-detection program. The following steps were used to determine if the two events occurred independently (see table): 1) The expected temporality if the two events occurred independently was calculated for interpeak intervals of three days (shortest interval) to eight days (longest interval); 2) The observed temporality (number of days from an FSH peak to the nearest wave emergence) was determined for each interpeak interval; and 3) The means for the expected and observed were compared by univariate *t*-tests. The expected temporality was calculated separately for each interval by calculating the average number of days between an FSH peak value and the nearest wave emergence if each day of wave emergence had equal probability of falling on any day between FSH peaks. The calculated expectancies are shown. The null hypothesis was that the difference between the expected day of occurrence and the observed day of occurrence was zero. In this data set, the mean number of observed days (0.3±0.2) from a peak to follicle emergence was shorter ($P<0.01$) than the expected number of days (1.1±0.1). Thus, the hypothesis of temporality was supported.

Follicular Data

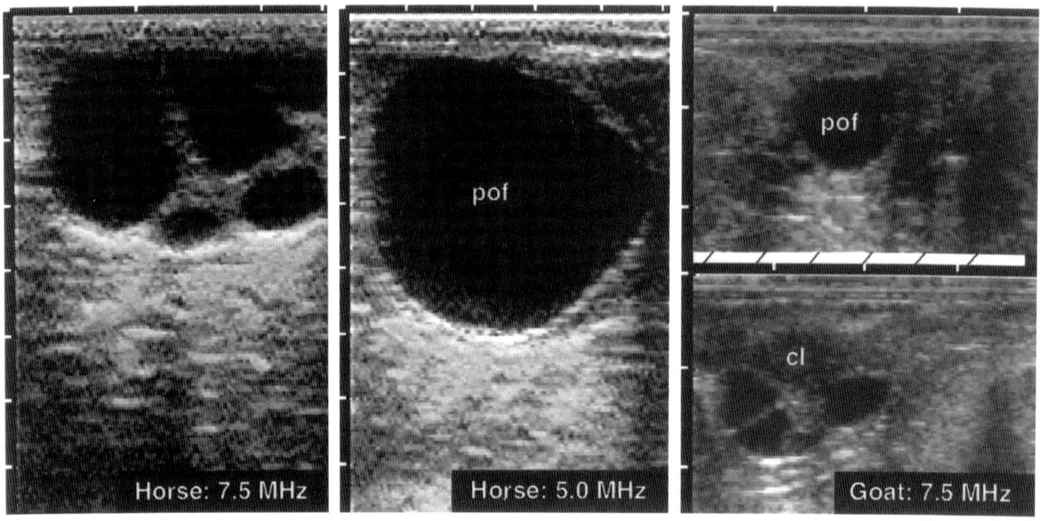

Ultrasonograms of ovaries from two species. cl=corpus luteum, pof=preovulatory follicle. Note the four small follicles beneath the goat corpus luteum. The diameters (left to right) are 6, 5, 2, and 6 mm.

Collection of follicular data is, by far, the most extensive, current research use of ultrasound in farm animals. Similar studies have apparently not been done in dogs and cats. Because ultrasonic derivation of follicular data is a new capability, scientists will need to devise creative statistical evaluation procedures. They will also need to develop clear, firm definitions with each writing until definitions become standardized. We are reaching the point where raw observations or individual profiles will no longer be adequate for scientific publication.

The phenomenon of growth of follicles in waves or cohorts in cattle and horses was initially accepted on the basis of inspection of ultrasonically derived follicular profiles. However, some waves may not be obvious by inspection and, furthermore, as new species are studied, the question of the presence or absence of waves may be perplexing. This fundamental question deserves a probability footing the same as other variable biological events. Goodness-of-fit, chi square methodologies, based on expectancy distributions if follicles emerged at random, for example, should be applied *(for an example, see 77)*.

The day of emergence of a follicular wave is an example of a reference point or end point that requires firm definition. Apparently, at the time of response to a stimulus, follicles may be at different diameters (e.g., 1 to 4 mm), and therefore the time when they attain a predesignated size may encompass many days *(heifers, 75; mares, 63)*. The day of emergence of a follicular wave, day of divergence in diameter between the dominant and subordinate follicles, day of attainment of growth cessation, maximum diameter, or regression of designated follicles can be used as reference points for testing hypotheses, for characterizing follicular waves *(63)*, and for studying temporal associations between events, such as follicle emergence and FSH release. Examples of reported definitions of the day of wave emergence include the day the retrospectively identified dominant follicle was 15 mm in mares *(14)* or 4 or 5 mm in heifers *(75)*, and the day of the lowest mean preceding a significant increase in diameter of the six largest follicles in mares *(67)*. The day of divergence, growth cessation, or regression can be based on a predeveloped definition requiring a minimal diameter criterion or change.

Another example of a statistical maneuver that seems simple—but isn't—is the comparison of follicular growth rates within or among waves. Firm, objective criteria are needed for selection of the days to be used, since for some follicles the growth rate may change dramatically as maximum diameter is approached.

Measurement or estimation of antral diameter also is subject to error and bias. The interface of the follicular fluid and the inner follicular wall provide the most distinct demarcation. Placement of the cursors should be standardized and consistent. Calibration can be done by measuring objects of known diameter with a phantom or in a water bath; the placement required to obtain the expected value should be noted. Some scanners are calibrated so the vertical or horizontal line of the cursor is placed next to the image of the tissue object rather than on it.

Maintaining day-to-day identity of follicles may not be accomplished if the operator attempts to physically measure every follicle. Therefore, estimations of diameters, especially of smaller follicles, may be preferred. Examination of data derived by estimation may disclose that the operator "did not like" certain diameters; there may be plenty of 10s, 12s and 15s but few 11s or 13s. Diameters can be subconsciously tilted toward compatibility with the hypothesis. The above caveats illustrate that a researcher's objectivity is challenged during the collection and evaluation of follicular ultrasound data.

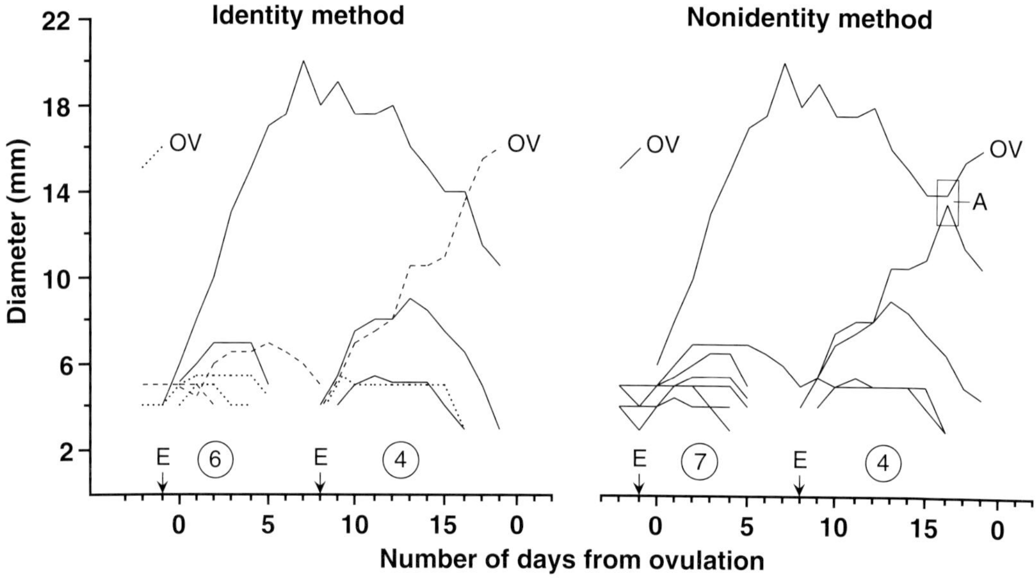

Day	Follicle diameters (mm)					
-2	15	5	4	4	4	4
-1	**16**	5	4	4	4	3
0	6	5	5	5	5	4
1	8	6	5.5	5	5	4.5
2	10	7	6	5.5	5	4
3	13	7	6.5	5.5	5	4
4	15	7	6.5	5.5	5	3
5	17	7	5	4.5	4	
6	17.5	6.5				
7	20	6				
8	18	5	4			
9	19	5.5	5.5			
10	17.5	7.5	7	5.5	4	
11	17.5	8	7.5	5	5	
12	18	8	8	5.5	5	
13	16	10.5	9	5	5	
14	15	10.5	8.5	5	5	
15	14	11	7.5	5	5	
16	14	13.5	6.5	5	4	
17	15.5	11.5	5	3	3	
18	**16**	10.5	4.5			

Identity and nonidentity methods in cattle. The identity method (upper left) involves maintaining the identity of individual follicles from day to day *(61)*. A sketch of each ovary is drawn for each day. Identified follicles are given a letter or other designation on the sketch, retrospectively, when first identified, and for as long as the follicle can be followed. The position of follicles relative to each other and the corpus luteum are used for identification. Bias is a real and continuing threat. It may be best not to profile the follicles on a graph until the study is completed; this may minimize the tendency to have follicles follow a preconceived path.

If treatment groups are involved, the sonographer should operate without knowledge of group and preferably without knowledge of the hypothesis being tested. For an instantaneous panoramic impression, the follicles can be profiled as shown. The number in circles is the number of follicles in each wave for this two-wave interovulatory interval. Depending on the research need, the target for identity and profiling can be set at any diameter. For some purposes, for example, it may be necessary to identify from day to day only follicles ≥ 7mm.

Another approach is to videotape the ultrasonic examinations for later evaluation. A separate videotape should be used for each ovary and each animal; this facilitates reference to the previous day's scan to help maintain a similar transducer-to-ovary orientation and to identify individual follicles. Practicing the technique before beginning an experiment will minimize the tendency to scan too rapidly.

In the nonidentity method, follicles are profiled on the basis of diameter without regard to day-to-day identity. Each follicle diameter for each day in each ovary can be tabulated on the basis of decreasing diameter from largest to smallest as shown in the table. Columns of data are then highlighted, ending at ovulation or when the data became discontinuous as shown in the table. The bold number indicates the diameter of the preovulatory follicle on the day before ovulation. Columns can be used only for data in which at least one follicle in a column is ≥4.5 mm or some other designated diameter. Each column of data is used to construct a continuous line of profiled data as shown in the figure (upper right). The dominant and subordinate follicles are identifiable from the profiles. When the profiles for successive dominant follicles involve opposite ovaries, their individual profiles can be drawn directly. When successive dominant follicles involve the same ovary, the profiles are interrupted on the days that the profiles for the two follicles cross. On the figure, the letter "A" has been used to designate the area of ambiguity. Often, however, the path followed by the two dominant follicles is evident even when on the same ovary. The day of emergence of a follicular wave is made on the basis of inspection of the profiles and is defined, for example, as the last day a group of follicles was 4 mm as indicated by subsequent increasing diameters. When an appropriate 4-mm follicle has not been detected, the lines can be visually projected retrospectively to 4 mm. When emergence of the cohort of follicles involves more than one day, the day of emergence can be defined by the first follicle to grow above 4 mm. The number of follicles per wave is determined with the aid of the columned data, since the profiling lines sometimes overlap, obscuring the number of follicles.

No difficulty has been experienced in identifying the day of wave emergence by the nonidentity method, even in pregnant heifers with development of successive dominant follicles in one ovary. The nonidentity method may be inadequate for distinguishing the plateau phase when one ovary is inactive. This may be especially so during pregnancy, since, unlike the estrous cycle, follicle identification will not be aided by the occurrence of ovulation. The method may also be inadequate for characterizing the dominant follicle when experimental treatments or pathologic processes profoundly alter the diameter profiles.

The nonidentity method seems suitable for studying the characteristics of dominant follicles (e.g., maximal diameter attained, rate of growth and regression). Follicular data can be collected more quickly and with less skill by the nonidentity method than by the identity method, and bias due to inspecting previous data, as required in the identity method, can be eliminated. The method should be suitable for studying the characteristics of follicular waves and the temporal relationships among follicles and other variables (e.g., FSH concentrations). Objectivity can be maintained by evaluating the waves without knowledge of treatment groups or other factors under study, but this precaution is applicable also to the identity method.

A combination of the identity and nonidentity methods also may be appropriate, especially when information on the profiles of the dominant follicle is crucial. For example, identity data can be collected for profiling follicles >7 mm, and nonidentity data can be collected to determine days of wave emergence and number of follicles per wave. In this way, the areas of ambiguity in the dominant follicle profiles can be minimized. In conclusion, the nonidentity method provides adequate criteria for determining days of emergence of a wave but cannot be used to locate the day of emergence of individual follicles. Day of divergence and the subsequent growth profile of the dominant follicle can be determined by either the nonidentity or identity methods.

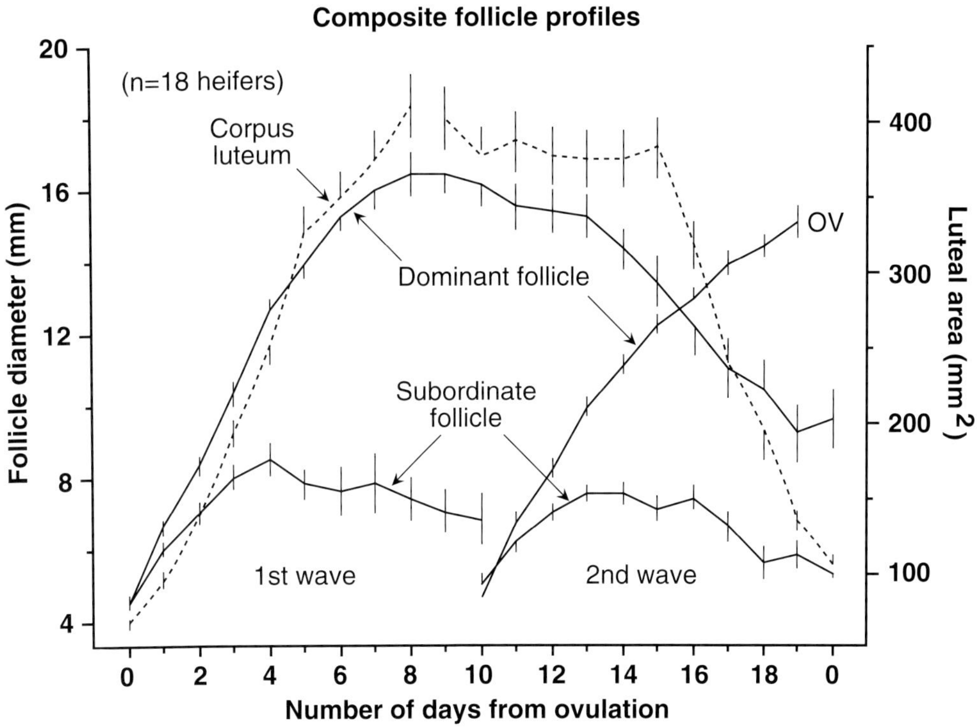

Mean profiles of ovarian structures in cattle. Data are from 18 cattle with two-wave interovulatory intervals *(75)*. The lengths of the interovulatory intervals were normalized (pg 154). The mean day of emergence (defined as attainment of 4 mm) for the dominant follicle and for the largest subordinate follicle for each wave were then centralized (pg 154) onto the normalized day scale. The normalization and centralization procedures permitted an average characterization of the components of waves and statistical analyses of events. This general approach of normalization and centralization is applicable to other species but requires the development of definition of waves and days of emergence.

Antral diameter (or mean diameter if the follicle is irregular) is our preferred end point; it seems easier to relate to diameter than to cross-sectional area or to calculated volume. However, as shown in the figure, we often use maximum cross-sectional area for the corpus luteum, so that central, nonluteinized areas can be subtracted from the total. This cannot be done meaningfully with diameters.

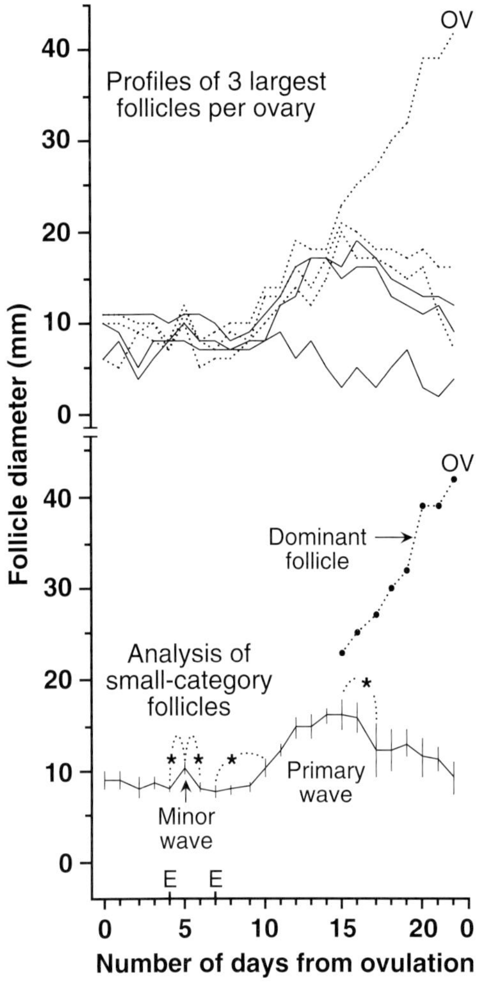

Mathematical method for detecting follicular waves in mares *(63,68)*. Initially (top panel), the diameters of the three largest follicles per ovary were profiled (dotted lines=left ovary; solid lines=right ovary). After the dominant follicle became identifiable, it was removed from the data set. The remaining six largest follicles per mare (lower panel; small category follicles) were analyzed for waves as indicated by a significant increase in diameter followed by a significant decrease. The minor wave is indicated by the absence of a dominant follicle, whereas the major wave gave origin to a dominant follicle. E=day of emergence of a wave as indicated by the nadir preceding a significant increase. OV=ovulation.

The mathematical approach eliminates bias resulting from inspecting data from the previous day, a requirement in the identity method; it also identifies waves earlier and with greater objectivity and uses the advantages of probability values. The mathematical method in mares has detected waves at mean follicle diameters of 9 to 12 mm in various studies and at means of 2 to 4 days earlier than for the identity method. The presence of minor waves of follicles was substantiated by ranking the largest follicles in all statistically detected waves from largest to smallest. The greatest discontinuity in decreasing diameters occurred between 34 and 28 mm. This difference (6 mm) was more than 4 standard deviations from the mean difference. The ranked data were therefore accepted as representing two populations of waves (largest follicle in major waves, 34 to 45 mm; in minor waves, 19 to 28 mm). Currently in mares, we routinely record the six largest follicles per ovary so that the data can be evaluated mathematically.

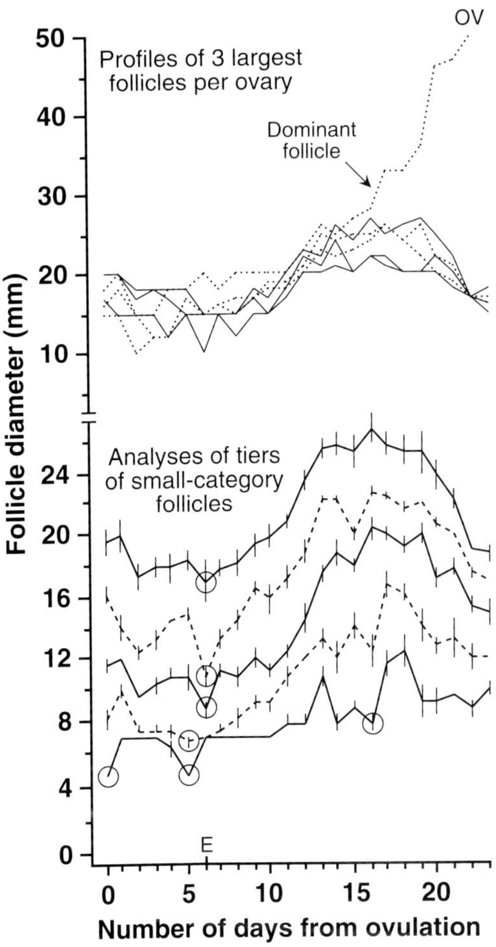

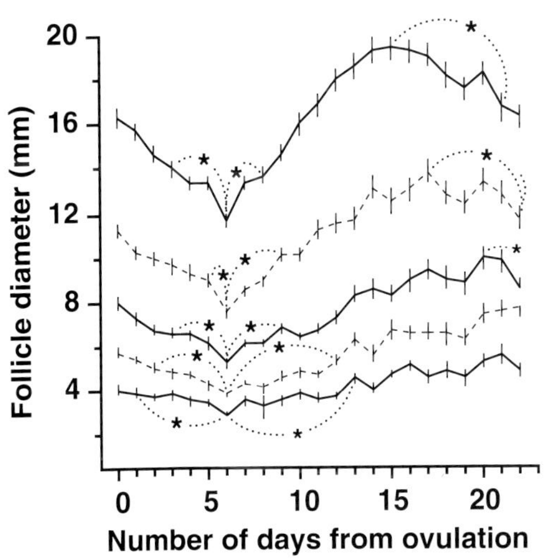

Tier method *(69)*. For each day and each mare, the follicles were combined for both ovaries (excluding identifiable dominant follicles) and were ranked from largest to smallest without regard to the day-to-day identity of individual follicles. The follicles were then divided into tiers of six follicles per tier (Tier 1, six largest follicles; Tier 2, six next-largest follicles, etc.). The follicles of each tier were analyzed by the mathematical method, as described on the facing page. The days of emergence of waves (significant increase followed by a significant decrease) are shown (indicated by a ring). A primary follicular wave was identified in all of 15 mares using Tier 1 for identification (E=day of emergence). The presence of underlying follicular waves (waves in Tiers 2 to 5) suggested that even follicles as small as 3 to 4 mm are involved in the wave phenomenon.

Composite data for 15 mares are shown in the lower panel *(69)*. Data for all tiers were centralized to six days after ovulation, the mean day of emergence of the ovulatory wave as determined from Tier 1. Significant differences are shown by asterisks. This approach has been used to show the time associations between development of follicles and changes in FSH concentrations *(69)*.

Computer-generated End Points

Ultrasonic image information may be digitized and analyzed by computer. Digitization is a procedure in which each pixel of an image is assigned a numeric value for brightness and location. Conversion of image information to numerical data allows the use of quantitative statistics for temporal characterizations or testing of hypotheses *(165, 167)*. However, the sophisticated processing does not eliminate bias. The operator retains the responsibility of selecting and delineating the areas that are to be processed, and these decisions are notoriously subject to bias. Computer analyses, therefore, can be dangerous and lull the operator into a false sense of well-being. Since it may not be practical to expose the computer set-up to barn conditions, the image information may be stored with a high resolution videotape system (pg 122). The analogue format used on the videotape is then reconverted to the digitized format at the laboratory.

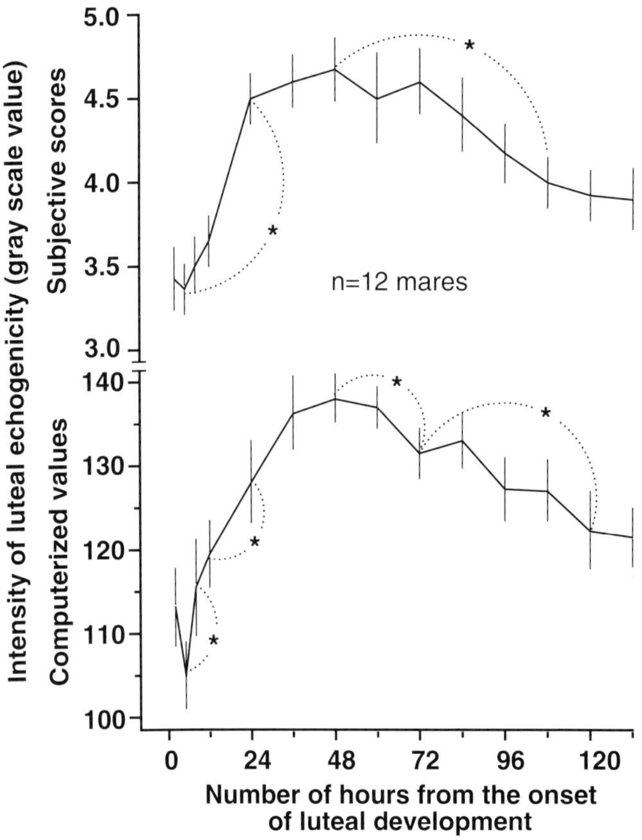

Pixel analysis of echogenicity *(167)*. The intensity of echogenicity of luteal tissue beginning two hours after ovulation was determined using two approaches. The first approach was a categorical technique in which luteal echogenicity was assigned a gray-scale score between 1 and 8 according to an eight-section gray-scale display located next to the image. Only the luteinized areas of the gland were evaluated for gray-scale echogenicity.

The second approach was a quantitative technique using digital image analysis or pixel analysis to examine luteal-gland tissue. Selected frames of real-time imaging were captured from videotape using a computer-operated frame grabber. The pixels comprising the ultrasound images were assigned numeric digits for brightness and location coordinates by the computer (digitization). Thus digitized, the images could be analyzed for shape, size, or echogenicity. A custom-made computer program was used, since appropriate commercial programs were not available at the time of the study; programs are now available (pg 168). In this study, images of the luteinized portion of the glands were analyzed for echogenicity. The outer borders of the luteal gland and central fluid pockets (nonechogenic areas) within the gland were traced with a computer mouse. Image information beyond the luteal gland border and within the central fluid area were deleted. The computer then generated a frequency table that provided mean gray-scale information for the pixels comprising the image of the luteal tissue.

The results of pixels analysis in assessing the intensity of luteal echogenicity closely paralleled the more subjective, visual results of gray-scale scoring. The increase in luteal echogenicity was first significant by 24 hours, using both approaches. Only a slight difference in the time interval was detected when luteal echogenicity first significantly declined (72 vs 108 hours by pixel analysis and scoring, respectively). The echogenicity changes were pronounced enough to be recognized using the eight zone gray-scale scoring system, and the operator's subjective evaluations were consistent. However, the pixel analysis approach should minimize potential inconsistencies within and among operators and provides an objective, quantitative approach. Area and shape of echogenicity of imaged structures may also be estimated using the pixel analysis technique (pg 164). Of the three measures, echogenicity is probably the most difficult to quantitate subjectively. Pixel analysis is capable of analyzing up to 256 shades of gray, whereas only 8 to 16 shades of gray are reasonably estimated using a subjective approach. In the use of ultrasound scanners for research, objectivity is important because the generated information depends upon image interpretation. A quantitative approach to estimating subtle echogenicity changes in tissue may be useful not only in reproduction, but also in other biological areas that use ultrasonography.

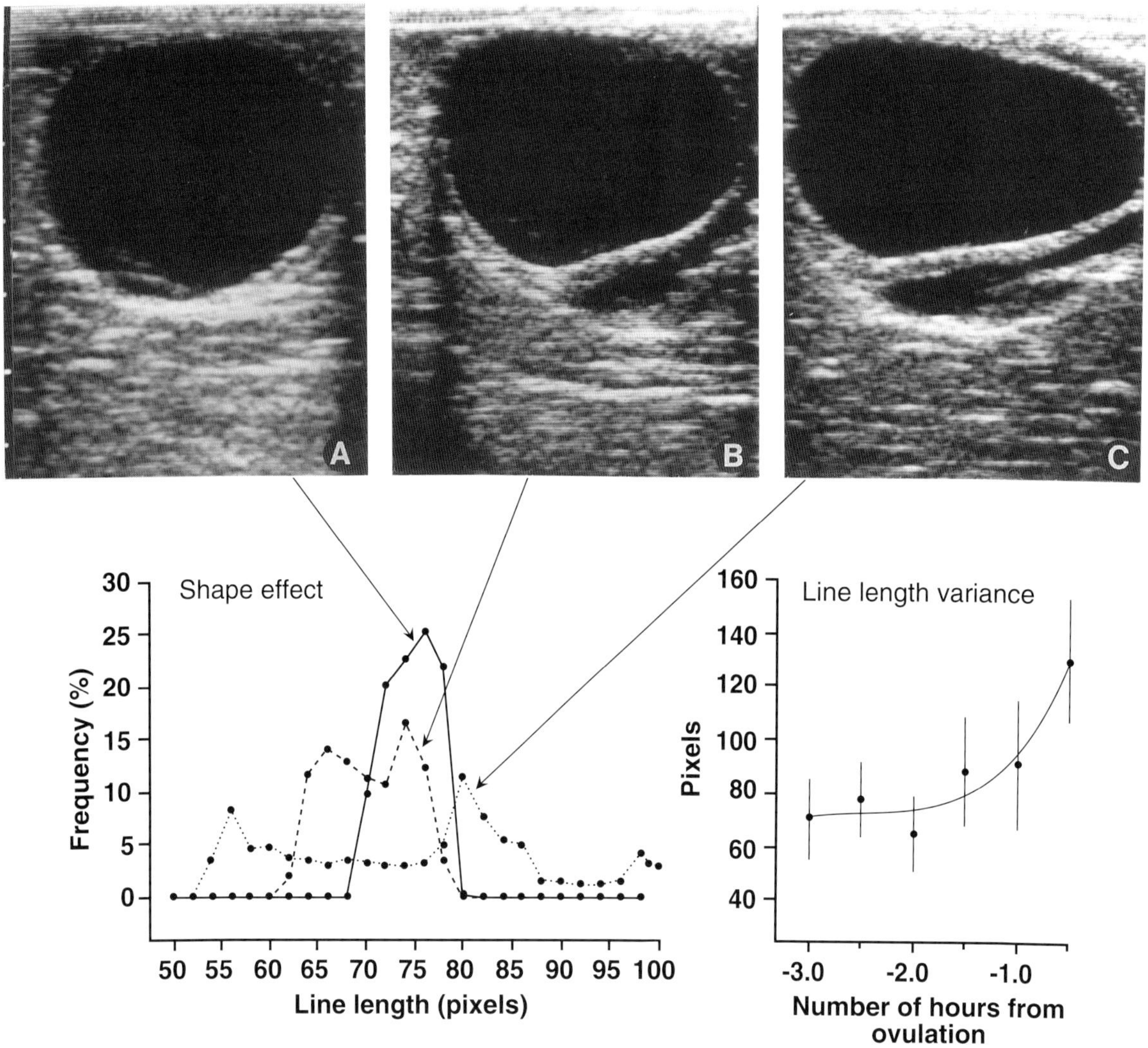

Use of pixel analyses to quantify changes in shape. Changing shapes of preovulatory equine follicles as determined by pixel analysis are shown *(165)*:

(A) A circular image taken 24 hours before ovulation.

(B) A semi-circular image taken at 2 hours and 17 minutes before ovulation.

(C) An oblong image taken 23 minutes before ovulation.

To quantify shape changes, a pixel analysis program was developed. A 16 MHz-386, IBM-AT compatible computer equipped with a high resolution video monitor, two megabytes random access memory, and 40 megabyte hard drive were used. The first step involved transferring the follicle images from videotape as digitized information to the computer using a frame-grabber board. The digitized images had a resolution of 512 x 480 pixels, with each pixel capable of representing up to 256 gray levels. A single image was selected for digitization from each three-minute taping of the largest cross-sectional area of the follicle. The selected image was the cross-sectional antral area with the apparent greatest deviation from circular during the three-minute taping. Selected images were assigned random numeric codes and subsequently stored in the computer memory. The computer-stored images were sequentially retrieved for pixel analysis according to numeric code. The operator was not aware of time of examination or animal identification during the pixel analysis procedure. Computer software was custom-designed to measure distances from the center of the antrum to the perimeter. The tissue interface between the antrum and follicle wall of a digitized image was traced with a computer mouse. All image information outside the traced area was deleted. The theoretical center of the antrum was calculated by the computer, based on the total pixel count within the traced antral area. Line distances radiating from the calculated center of the antrum to each pixel at the traced perimeter of the antrum were calculated. The line lengths were measured in terms of the number of pixels traversed by a line (approximately 3.7 pixels/mm). For example, a follicle with a circular cross-sectional image, a radius of 20 mm, and a circumference of 126 mm would involve approximately 466 radial line lengths (circumference x 3.7 pixels/mm) with a mean line length of 74 pixels (radius x 3.7 pixels/mm).

The size of each follicle was measured by mean and median line-lengths in pixels, and shape was quantified by the magnitude of line-length variance. Line-length variance was calculated by squaring the standard deviation of line lengths for each follicle. Thus, increasing variances represented increasing departures from the circular shape. The spread of the line-length distribution changed as the follicles changed shape from circular to oblong. Preovulatory-follicle shape, as expressed by line-length variance, differed significantly among examinations (right panel); the regression line that best characterized the data is shown. The increase in line-length variance was attributed to a gradual flattening of the cross-sectional image of the antrum from circular to oblong as ovulation approached.

Recent abstracts *(121, 163)* indicate that studies have begun on computer-assisted analysis of ultrasonic images of dominant follicles in heifers. Apparently, reviews will be published in Theriogenology (Issue 1, 1995).

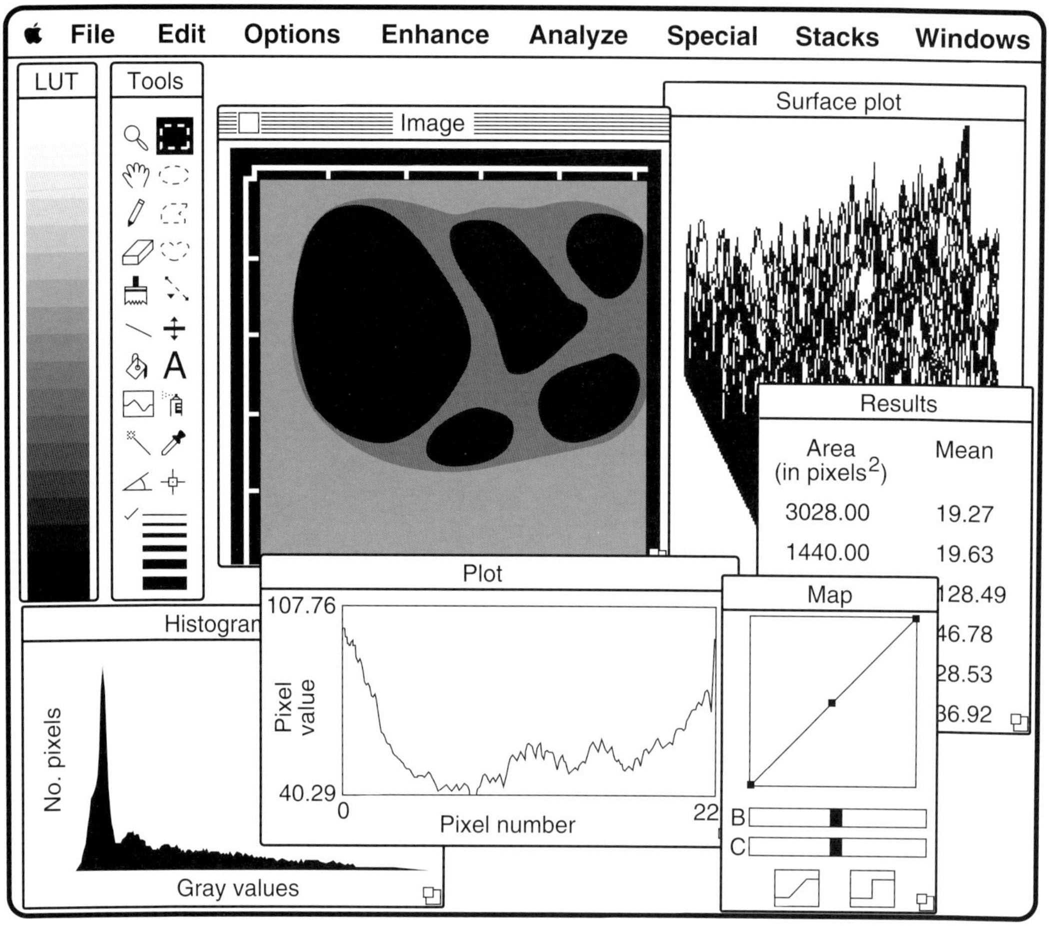

NIH Image program. The figure shows examples of window displays for measurements and profile plots and a simulated image of an equine ovary. The tools window is for making selections for editing, drawing, and measuring. The map window is for adjusting image contrast and brightness and for thresholding. This image analysis system for Macintosh computers is available from the National Institutes of Health without charge; it is in the public domain. The program and instruction manual can be obtained immediately by Internet users by electronic mail (source information: pg 197). The program can acquire, display, edit, enhance, analyze, and print ultrasound images. It reads and provides compatibility with many other programs, including those for scanning, processing, editing, publishing, and analyzing images. It supports many standard image-processing functions, including contrast enhancement, density profiling, smoothing, sharpening, edge detection, and median filtering. The NIH image program can be used to measure area, gray value, center, and angle of orientation of selected areas. Pixels (picture elements) are represented by 8-bit integers, ranging in value from 0 to 255. The image program follows the Macintosh convention and displays zero pixels with a value of zero as white and those with a value of 255 as black or vice versa. The system requires a Macintosh with at least 4 megabytes of memory. We use a Quadra 840AV (pg 126). The monitor must have the ability to display 256 shades of gray. Other work stations and software systems are available *(12)*.

M-mode Imaging

A research tool that apparently has not been used in reproductive biology of animals is M-mode (motion mode) imaging (pg 23). The most obvious application of this modality in reproductive biology is the determination of embryonal and fetal heart rate. The path to be examined is marked with a cursor line on a real-time B-mode image, and the designated slice is then evaluated by M-mode. Unfortunately, probe movement (from mare or operator) and independent fetal movement can be challenging and result in a "smeared" M-mode image. However, the B-mode image can be monitored in real time to help maintain or relocate the proper slice until a readable M-mode profile is obtained. Experimental error results from deviations in the precise position chosen for placement of the two cursor marks but probably (not tested) is no greater than the experimental error resulting from counting beats and using a stop watch. Possible research and clinical uses of the fetal-heart monitoring technique have not been explored, and other uses of M-mode in animal reproductive biology have not been identified. An example of M-mode evaluation of the fetal heart is shown on the next page.

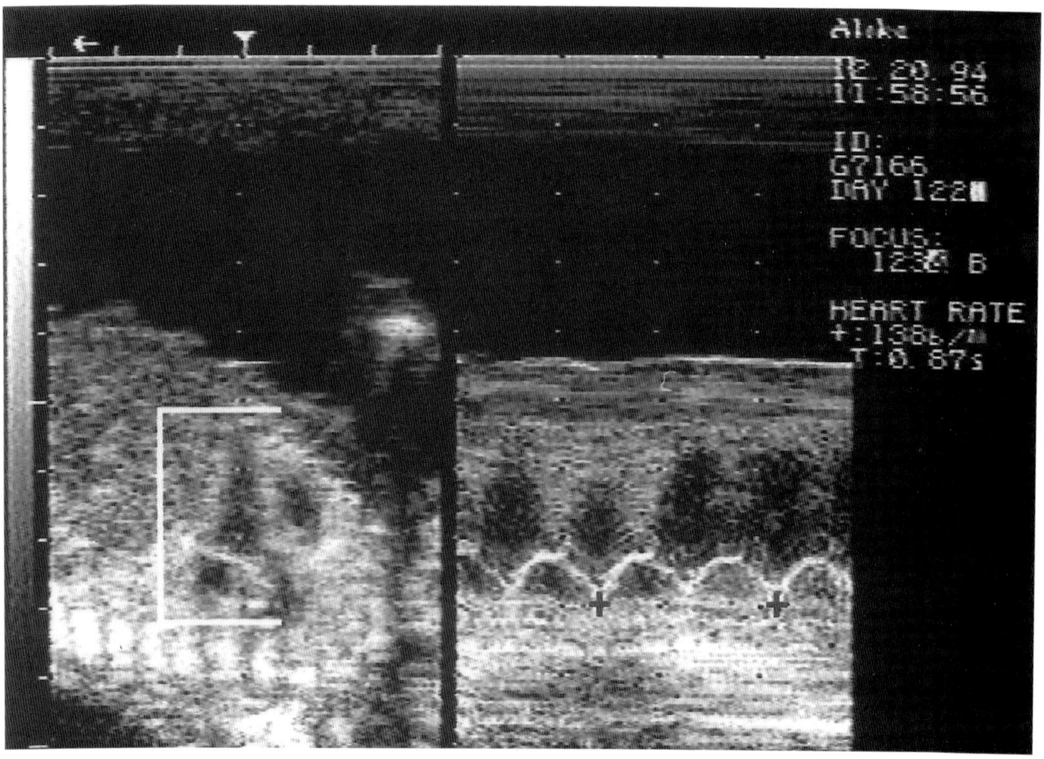

M-Mode display of fetal heartbeats. In this example, the B-mode image of an equine fetal heart at Day 122 is shown on the left; the heart is indicated by the bracket. An M-mode cursor line was placed over the beating heart on the real-time B-mode image and is depicted by the vertical row of dots. The cursor line represents the slice that will be sampled for the M-mode image (right panel). The vertical axis of the M-mode sonogram represents depth and the horizontal axis represents time. The time interval between each vertical row of dots is 0.5 seconds. The changing depths resulting from the beating heart are represented by the rhythmic lines on the M-mode image. Note the echogenic undulating line from the division between heart chambers, the alternating anechoic and echogenic areas resulting from an open and closed beating ventricle (above the undulating echogenic line) and images from the atrium (below the line). The heart rate is calculated by the scanner's computer system based on the distance (time) between two heart cycles or beats; two cursor marks (black crosses) have been placed on the image to identify two cycles. The measured time interval (0.87 seconds) and the computed heart rate (138 beats/minute) are displayed.

Part Four

SUMMARY

Chapter 10

SUMMARY

NOTE: Pages with detailed information are given throughout the summary.

1. Introduction (pgs 7 to 26)

Gray-scale diagnostic ultrasonography is a method for noninvasive visualization of the internal anatomy of the reproductive organs and their payload—the conceptus (pg 7). High-frequency sound waves are used to produce images of soft tissues of internal organs (pg 8). In the large species, transrectal scanning is used with the transducer held in the rectum directly over the organs of interest. In the small species, the transabdominal route can be used. Electric current is applied to crystals in the transducer, producing vibrations characteristic of the crystals and resulting in sound waves. The operator directs the sound waves through the tissues by moving or varying the angle of the transducer as desired. The short distance from the contact area (rectal wall, skin) to the viewing area allows the use of high-frequency scanners that produce images with much detail. The sound beams that pass through the tissues are quite thin (e.g., 2 mm in the focal zone), and a thin "slice" of tissue is sampled. The two-dimensional image seen on the screen is analogous to a histologic section (pg 9).

Tissues have different abilities to either propagate or reflect sound waves. The proportion of the sound waves that is reflected is received by the transducer, converted to electric impulses, and displayed as an echo on the ultrasound screen. The characteristics of various tissue interfaces determine what proportion of the sound waves will be reflected. The reflected portion is represented on the ultrasound image by shades of gray, extending from black to white. Liquids (follicular fluid, yolk sac fluid) do not reflect sound waves and are said to be anechoic or nonechogenic; therefore, the image of a liquid-containing structure appears black on the screen. At the other extreme, dense tissues (cervix, fetal bone) reflect more of the sound waves and appear white on the screen. Such tissues are said to be echogenic. Other tissues are seen in various shades of gray depending upon their echogenicity or ability to reflect sound waves.

Modern ultrasound instruments for examining the reproductive tracts of animals are B-mode, real-time scanners. B-mode refers to brightness modality, in which the ultrasonic imaging is a two-dimensional display of dots. The brightness of the dots is proportional to the amplitude of the returning echoes. Real-time imaging refers to the "live" or moving display in which the echoes are recorded continuously, and events such as fetal leg movements and heartbeat can be observed as they occur. Some scanners have videotaping capabilities so that the moving images can be preserved. They may be played back through the ultrasound scanner or a television set. The moving image also can be "frozen" to facilitate measurements or photographic reproduction.

Clinical need was the first impetus for the marketing of scanners in the animal field (pg 11). Creative clinical applications of real-time sonography continue to be reported. Clinical uses include determining the reproductive status of the ovaries and uterus; diagnosing solitary and multiple pregnancies; diagnosing fetal sex, embryonic loss, fetal viability, and pathology of the ovaries and the tubular organs; and estimating fetal age.

The history of ultrasonography began with the discovery of the piezoelectric effect of certain crystals in 1880 (pg 18). The principles of ultrasonic detection were refined in World War II for locating submarines. The development of gray-scale imaging and real-time imaging in the 1970s constituted major breakthroughs in the adaptability of ultrasound to the biological fields. The technology of B-mode, real-time imaging was first used in animals in 1980.

Ultrasonography is rapidly becoming established as a superb, potentially revolutionary, research tool (pg 20). In the short time that ultrasonic imaging has been used in research, many discoveries have resulted, some of which would otherwise have escaped detection for many years. Included among these discoveries are the following: 1) the phenomena of embryo mobility and fixation in mares; 2) the mechanism of natural embryo reduction in mares; 3) the natural uncurling of the uterine horns during estrus in heifers and llamas; 4) the incidental, rather than obligatory, formation of the corpus hemorrhagicum in mares; 5) the differential patterns of uterine contractility in mares and cattle during the estrous cycle and corresponding days of pregnancy; 6) the patterns of follicular evacuation in mares; 7) the precise nature of growth and regression of individual follicles in cattle, goats, horses, sheep, and llamas; 8) resurgence in growth of the primary corpus luteum in association with the release of equine chorionic gonadotropin; and 9) expulsion of conceptus debris through the cervix after embryonic death in cattle and horses rather than elimination by resorption.

2. Waves and Echoes (pgs 27 to 35)

The origin of audible sound from a drumhead, traveling of the resulting waves through air, echoing of the waves from a mountainside, reception of the echoes by ear drums, and processing of the eardrum vibrations by the internal auditory system are comparable to the origin of ultrasound from transducer crystals, traveling of the resulting waves through tissue, echoing of the waves from tissue reflectors, reception of the echoes by the transducer crystals, and processing of the crystal vibrations by the ultrasound scanner (pg 28). Diagnostic ultrasound originates from piezoelectric crystals that expand and contract when subjected to an electric current and, conversely, produce an electric current when compressed by returning echoes. Crystal expansion causes compression of neighboring tissue molecules, and contraction causes decompression similar to the response of air molecules to a vibrating drumhead. In this way, the ultrasound waves travel through tissue. The delay between origin of the waves and reception of the echoes is used to determine the distance from the crystals to the reflector.

A wavelength is the distance encompassed by an area of compression and the accompanying area of decompression and is depicted as a sine wave (pg 28). Frequency refers to the number of vibrations of the sound source (ultrasound crystals) per second and is measured in hertz (Hz) units. One hertz is one cycle per second and a megahertz (MHz) is one million cycles per second. Ultrasound is defined as any sound with a frequency of more than 20,000 Hz. Frequencies used for transrectal examination of the reproductive tract of animals are 3.0 to 7.5 MHz. Speed or velocity is the time required for a wavelength to pass a given point. In soft biological tissue, ultrasound waves travel at an average speed of 1540 meters/second.

Attenuation is the progressive weakening of the ultrasound waves as they travel through tissue, thereby limiting the depth of penetration (pg 32). The heterogeneous nature of tissues results in tissue interfaces wherever tissues of different acoustic properties are in contact. When sound waves cross an interface, a portion is returned to the transducer in the form of a reflection or echo. The magnitude of the difference in acoustic impedance between the tissues on each side of the interface determines how much of the waves will be reflected. Usually only a small amount is reflected, and the remainder is available to interact with other interfaces deeper in the tissue mass. The difference in impedance is sometimes so great that most of the wave is reflected. For this reason, one cannot "see" through a soft tissue and air interface. This occurs commonly in ultrasonic examination of the reproductive tract due to air pockets in the intestines (pg 33). Air is also a troublesome barrier when trapped between the crystals and the tissue being examined. For this reason, an acoustic coupler or gel may be applied between the crystals and the contact surface.

Refraction refers to the bending of the sound waves as they cross tissues or fluids with different acoustic properties. This is comparable to the bending of a light beam as it passes from air into water. Refraction is a common cause of an artifact in which a distinct shadow appears below the lateral edges of spherical fluid-filled structures. Scatter occurs when a sound wave encounters an interface that is irregular or smaller than the wavelength. Scatter is very important in imparting ultrasonic textures that are characteristic for a given tissue.

For production of ultrasound pulses, transducer crystals are subjected to a short series of electric excitations, resulting in a short series of vibrations (pg 34). As a result, a well-defined burst or pulse of waves is produced that travels through a gel coupler and into the medium. The short, pulsed nature of the generated waves allows an interval of quiescence to permit reception of potential echoes by the same crystals (pg 35). For example, the pulse of waves may be 2 to 3 mm in length and contain four cycles. The frequency of ultrasound crystals is so great that 1,000 pulses, each consisting of three or four cycles, may be emitted per second despite the requirement that there be a pause between pulses for echo detection. Higher-frequency crystals (e.g., 5.0 MHz) have the same number of waves per pulse, but the pulse is shorter than that of lower-frequency crystals (e.g., 3.0 MHz). These relationships are the basis for one of the tenets of ultrasound—higher frequency results in better resolution.

3. Sending and Receiving (pgs 37 to 50)

The crystals for sending sound waves into tissue and receiving the returning echoes are housed in a multicrystal assembly called the transducer or probe. Most of the ultrasound scanners for examination of the reproductive tracts in animals use linear-array systems (pg 38). Linear array refers to the side-by-side arrangement of the rectangular piezoelectric crystals along the transducer's length. The examining field and the two-dimensional image are rectangular. Sector and convex-array transducers are also used. Sector refers to the pie-shaped examining field and image. Intrarectal transducers are oriented primarily lengthwise with respect to the animal. The image obtained from a sector transducer can represent either a cross-sectional or longitudinal sample of tissue with respect to the body orientation, and the image from a linear-array transducer represents a longitudinal sample.

Linear-array transducers consist of 60 to 120 or more elements (crystals). Two of the current models of veterinary scanners utilize 64 elements (pg 41). Elements are fired in small clusters beginning at one end, and then the cluster format is moved in one-element increments along the length of the linear array (pg 42). For example, a cluster of elements 1, 2, 3, 4, 5, 6, and 7 may be fired. After the cluster is activated, the same cluster is used to detect the echoes by allowing suitable time for echo reception. Then the second cluster (elements 2 to 8) is fired by moving one step down the array. The sound field resulting from firing a cluster of elements is termed a beam (pg 44). Beams are imaginary; they merely outline the three-dimensional path followed by each pulse. A complete sweep of beams across all the elements in the array produces one image or frame. The use of frames permits real-time images—that is, images that move as the structures move. Detection of rapid movements requires rapid frame rates. Typical frame rates are 20 to 30 frames per second.

Resolution refers to the ability of an ultrasound pulse to distinguish between two closely spaced reflectors (pg 46). High-frequency transducers give better resolution, due to the relatively shorter pulses. Shorter pulses are less likely to overlap two neighboring reflecting surfaces. Focusing narrows a portion of the beam profile and thereby increases the amplitude of the echoes from reflectors at a certain depth (pg 47). Beams may be focused in the thickness plane to give better lateral resolution at a given depth. This is done by using curved crystals (internal focusing) or by placing an acoustic lens beneath the crystals (external focusing). By modifying the element-firing sequence, beams also can be focused in the width plane (electric focusing). With higher frequency transducers, the focal region is closer to the transducer. A 3.0 or 3.5 MHz transducer is more suited to studying the large postpartum uterus or a large fetus by either external or intrarectal placement of the transducer in large species or for transabdominal work in the small farm species. A 5.0 MHz transducer is more suited to detailed transrectal study of the reproductive tract or early conceptus in large species and for transabdominal studies in small species.

4. Processing (pgs 51 to 63)

Echoes from tissue reflectors are received by the piezoelectric crystals of the transducer. The electric signals generated by the crystals travel from the transducer to the ultrasound console through a coaxial cable. The echoes are initially processed by the receiver of the console, where the echo signal is amplified and compensation is made for loss of intensity due to attenuation (pg 52). The degree of amplification is called gain and is comparable to volume in the control of audible sound. The concept of gain must be thoroughly understood because proper adjustment of the gain controls is one of the most important variables under the continuous control of the ultrasonographer. On most scanners, near gain, far gain, and overall gain controls are provided for the near field, far field, and the overall image, respectively. Proper balancing of the controls is needed to provide maximum clarity at various depths and to minimize artifactual responses.

The scan converter stores the amplified signals and shows the resulting information on an echo display screen (pg 53). Modern animal scanners have digital scan converters that utilize the digital system that is used in personal computers. The scan converter records the echo information at an address that corresponds to the location of the echo source. The television display screen uses a similar address system, so that the addresses and the accompanying code for level of gray are read from the converter to the corresponding address on the television screen. The digital scan converter is also the major synchronizer in the system; the timing of events within the converter involves regulating the transducer scanning rate on one side and the television format on the other. Storage of the data representing signals provides the opportunity not only to see the completed image but also to manipulate the image into a preferred form. A manipulation done after the data are stored is called postprocessing and includes automatic electronic smoothing of the image. The gain controls are adjusted while viewing the echoes on the screen (pg 54). These controls allow the operator to compensate for attenuation by equalizing the echoes coming from different tissue depths. Proper adjustment of the gain controls is crucial in building a balanced and pleasant image.

The term B-mode refers to brightness modulation of the dots or pixels on the echo display screen. Each pixel or picture element corresponds to a location in the scan converter memory, which in turn corresponds to the location of a tissue reflector (pg 55). Echo signals are presented as brightened pixels with the distance from the top of the image to the pixel representing the distance from transducer to tissue reflector. The brightness of a pixel corresponds to the amplitude of that individual echo signal. Tissue reflectors or interfaces may reflect all of the sound pulse, resulting in very bright (white) pixels. Interfaces of intermediate reflectivity return only a portion of the pulse, resulting in gray pixels (pg 56). The terms hypoechogenic and hyperechogenic are sometimes used to describe low and high intensities of echogenicity, respectively. Brightness is represented by shades of gray extending from white (very bright or highly echogenic) to black (no discernible echo; nonechogenic).

Information in the scan converter is transferred to the echo-display screen (pg 58). Electrons ("cathode rays") are produced by heating a filament in the electron gun of the oscilloscope and are focused into a well-defined electron beam. The beam strikes the phosphor in the screen, causing it to emit light. The beam is directed across the screen by electric signals applied to the deflection plates. The pattern of movement of the electron beam across the viewing screen is called a raster scan. The scan pattern begins in the upper left corner of the screen, moves steadily across, snaps back, and then begins another line. The result is a pattern of movement over the screen that forms a sweep or set of horizontal raster lines. As the raster lines move across the screen, the electron beam turns on and off, thereby producing the vertical scanning lines (pg 59). Therefore, each point at which a raster line crosses a scanning line represents one pixel. The intensity of the electric signals originating from the memory of the scan converter provides the appropriate information for the intensity (gray-scale level) of the oscilloscope's electron beam for each pixel. Thus, the information stored at each address of the converter is transferred to each pixel of the viewing screen as the sweeping beam of electrons passes over the appropriate pixel. Digital systems are very fast, so that recording into the memory, modifying data, and transferring data to the screen can all be done without one process interfering with the other. The quality of engineering in the display system is a source of variation in image quality (pg 61). Part of the smoothness of the digital television image comes from the use of very small pixels. Some scanners in the animal market are undesirable because large pixels give the image a checkered appearance.

5. Interpreting (pgs 65 to 82)

Proper interpretation of the echoes on an ultrasound screen is crucial. Interpretation requires knowledge of the relationships between tissues and echoes and the ability to differentiate between true and artifactual responses (pg 65). There are two types of reflections (specular and nonspecular) which are presented as echoes on the screen and represent tissue structure. Certain tissue formations also cause waves to bend (refract), bounce back and forth or re-echo (reverberate), become weakened (attenuated) or entirely blocked. As a result, distortions appear on the ultrasound image which can be mistaken for normal or pathologic structures or changes. These artifactual echoes complicate the interpretation process. Artifacts are especially common during imaging of the reproductive tract because of the many pockets of bowel gas, fluid-filled structures, and the pelvic bone.

A specular reflection results when a pulse strikes an interface that is smooth, wider than the pulse, and parallel to the transducer (pg 66). Usually, only a small portion of the pulse that strikes such an interface is reflected. The major portion of the pulse continues past the interface as a transmitted pulse or beam. If the wall of the opposite side of an encapsulated, fluid-filled structure is smooth, the opposite wall also will act as a specular reflector. The specular reflection appears as a hyperechogenic echo on the viewing screen. Specular echoes are commonly seen on the upper and sometimes lower surfaces of fluid-filled spherical structures (e.g., uterine cysts, follicles, and equine embryonic vesicles). Nonspecular or diffuse reflections originate when a pulse strikes a rough interface or one that is narrower than the pulse (pg 68). When the ultrasound pulse strikes such a surface, the effective interfaces are narrower than the beam, and scatter of echoes occurs. The net result is a displayed pattern, texture, or speckling that may help to identify a given tissue. In contrast to specular reflectors, echo amplitude for nonspecular reflectors is not dependent on beam angle. Gray-scale imaging fully utilizes the scatter phenomenon of nonspecular or diffuse reflections. The bright and dark areas of a speckled image do not necessarily correspond to physical structures in the tissue. The speckled area is an interference pattern that nevertheless is representative of the organ or tissue and is called the tissue's echotexture.

A shadow artifact is caused by a noticeable decrease or absence of ultrasonic waves due to blockage or deviation of the sound beams (pg 70). Shadow artifacts appear as a black column beneath a very dense structure (e.g., bone) or beneath the lateral walls of fluid-filled structures. Reflection may be the entire cause of beam deviation when the acoustic properties are the same on both sides of the reflecting surface (e.g., side of ovary). However, if there is a mismatch of sound speed on the two sides, refraction occurs, which is similar to the bending of a light beam when it hits water. Enhancement or through-transmission artifacts are common in sonograms of the reproductive tract because of the presence of fluid-filled structures (pg 71). These artifacts result when the ultrasound beams pass through a reflector-free structure (e.g., fluid-filled). The beam is not depleted (attenuated) by echo production while passing through the fluid. Therefore, when the beam emerges from the far side, the amplitude of the pulse is greater than in the tissues on each side. The relatively greater amplitude or strength of the sound beams distal to the fluid-filled structure results in a column of relatively brighter echoes beneath the structure.

Reverberation is a process wherein an echo bounces between two strong interfaces until the ultrasound pulses are exhausted by attenuation (pg 74). The following three distinguishing features help identify reverberation artifacts: 1) they are equidistant, 2) they gradually diminish in intensity, and 3) they are oriented parallel to the reflective interface. If a very reflective interface is involved (soft tissue/gas), none of the pulse is transmitted through the interface (pg 75). Therefore, an acoustic shadow results and the reverberation echoes on the screen are placed in the shadow. Reverberation artifacts are very common in the pelvic area because of pockets of bowel gas.

Structures devoid of reflectors appear black (anechoic) on a properly adjusted viewing screen (pg 82). The requirement for nonechogenicity is uniformity of fluid or tissue makeup so that reflectors are absent or inconsequential. An example of an anechoic solid structure is the equine fetal hoof. Anechoic fluid-filled structures abound in the reproductive tract (e.g., follicle, placental sacs, uterine cysts, and physiologic and pathologic accumulations of fluid in the lumens of tubular genitalia). Fluid-filled structures are useful for adjusting scanner controls; the controls should be adjusted until the fluid areas are black but with minimal loss of information in the soft tissue areas.

6. Scanners (pgs 85 to 112)

Transducers for intrarectal use must be designed for ease of insertion and manipulation within the rectum and for minimization of trauma (pg 86). The difference in resolving power between a 3.5 MHz and 5.0 MHz transducer can be appreciated on a practical basis in the detectability of structures in the reproductive tract of large animals (pg 89). Capabilities of 3.5 and 5.0 MHz transducers, respectively, are as follows: 1) minimum diameter of detectable follicles—6 to 8 mm and 2 to 3 mm; 2) detectability of corpus luteum—from Day 0 to Day 5 and from Day 0 to regression; and 3) earliest detection of equine conceptus—Day 11 (6 to 7 mm) and Day 9 or 10 (3 to 4 mm). The distance from the transducer face to the center of the ovary or the lumen of a nongravid uterus is only a few centimeters. Therefore, a higher frequency transducer (e.g., 5.0 MHz) with a focal point of 3 or 4 cm is well suited for examination of the reproductive tract in nonpregnant or early pregnant animals. The lower frequency transducers (e.g., 3.5 MHz) are more suited for transrectally examining the uterus in large animals during late pregnancy or soon after parturition or for transabdominal imaging of the conceptus in the smaller farm species.

The console contains the components for coordinating pulse emission from the transducer, processing the signals from the transducer, and displaying the resulting image on a viewing screen (pg 93). Diagnostic ultrasound scanners therefore contain complex electronic circuitry. Despite the complexity of the console, it should be durable and require minimal servicing. Because the scanners may be used in barns, they should be designed to exclude as much dust and dirt as possible and should be readily cleaned. Most animal models have near, far, and overall gain controls; a magnification or zoom feature; a freeze button; brightness and contrast controls; electronic calipers; and a keyboard for making annotations on the image to permanently identify videotapes and photographs. Proper adjustments of the gain controls are crucial to building a balanced and pleasing image. The gain adjustments equalize the signal amplitude at various depths (pg 97). When the amplifier gain is too high, the echoes are too strong and the display is overloaded; conversely, if the gain is too low, the echoes are inadequate. Usually, the gain controls can be adjusted at the beginning of the examination of a number of animals with no adjustment thereafter except for occasional fine-tuning. All controls (brightness, contrast, gains) must be considered together. The adjustment of the brightness control, for example, directly influences the optimal setting for the gain controls.

Tissue-mimicking testers or phantoms can be used to monitor a scanner's continuing performance (pg 89). The phantoms contain test objects (e.g., nylon filaments or pins, fluid-filled cylinders) embedded in tissue-mimicking material. A baseline is established for each instrument (transducers and consoles) when it is new or at peak performance (pg 101). Characteristics considered in quality tests include depth of ultrasonic penetration, linear measurement accuracy (horizontal and vertical), resolution (axial and lateral), and the quality of fluid-filled structures. Lateral-resolution tests may utilize a vertical row of pins; images of the pins mimic the width and shape of the ultrasound beam, and measurements of the pin images indicate the changing resolutions at various depths. Axial resolution is tested by pins placed in a curve at varying distances.

The purchase of an ultrasound scanner is a major investment, so potential buyers are justified in thoroughly researching the purchase (pg 110). Makes and models of scanners vary widely in capabilities and incidental provisions. All individuals will desire high quality and good service, for example, but may differ in their general needs. This is especially true for clinical versus research requirements. Researchers may want elaborate provisions for annotations, measurements (e.g., area), photography and videotaping, and multiple freeze-frame memories. Clinicians may prefer less elaborate schemes, especially if it means a lower price and fewer breakdowns. A scanner should not, however, be selected on the basis of its specifications alone. For example, a scanner with many elements will provide poor quality if other aspects of the engineering (e.g., damping, electrical insulation) are poor. Good resolving power and penetrating capability are not assured on the basis of transducer frequency. Many other factors are involved. The most reliable information on quality is obtained from a personal trial under the potential buyer's conditions. An excellent criterion for evaluating the quality of a scanner centers on its ability to consistently image by transrectal examination a developing or mature corpus luteum in large animals (pg 112).

7. Hard Copy (pgs 113 to 127)

Hard copy is defined as the readable printed copy from a machine, such as a computer. In ultrasonography, the term is commonly used for photographs (sonograms) or videotapes of images (pg 113). Communication and documentation of results are important aspects of ultrasonography. Specialized instruments and knowledge are required to produce high-quality hard copy, whether a Polaroid image for a mare owner's scrapbook or a set of images for a professional or scientific publication. The preparation of projection slides and videotapes is very useful, if not a requirement, for educational purposes, both for the clinician and researcher. Consideration should be given to the following: 1) Polaroid photography (pg 114), a rapid but expensive approach used by veterinarians; 2) negative-based photography, including organization of files and record keeping (pg 117); 3) preparation of slides for projection (pg 121); and 4) production of videotapes and preparation of photographs from videotapes (pg 122). In the production of photographs, a freeze-frame memory on the scanner is used. The quality of the photographs depends upon the quality of the real-time images and the quality of the freeze-frame provision, as well as the quality of photographic instrumentation and technique.

In recent years, video printers have become available for immediate production of high-quality prints (pg 120). In the more expensive printers, color and black-and-white prints are produced in publication quality. The input video signal is digitally processed in frame memory so that 1 to 4 images can be printed on one 100 x 140 mm print. It takes about 80 seconds to output a print. Less expensive printers are available and are adequate if only black-and-white copy is needed. Such printers produce a high-quality print in only a few seconds for less than 10¢ per copy.

Ultrasonic scanners can be integrated with computers, as well as with tape recorders and printers (pg 125). A system that will take images from a video source and store them in a personal computer is being marketed for animal work. Examples of uses include enhancing, enlarging, filtering, colorizing, preparing slides or prints, and transmitting images by telephone. Other computer-videotape work stations are available.

8. Techniques (pgs 130 to 144)

Attainment of the maximum capabilities of the instruments requires not only proper adjustments of the controls, but also good scanning techniques (pg 129). The operator must develop a thorough and realistic mental impression of the anatomy and orientation of the organs. Orientation is especially important in transrectal imaging of the uterus and ovaries because of their mobility. Although modern veterinary ultrasound scanners for large animals are portable, they provide much incentive for the development of a centralized examining area on farms (pg 135). A platform or cabinet can be built immediately next to the rear of the restraining chute. The height of the platform should position the scanner so that the screen and controls are approximately at eye level. The scanner should be close to the chute so that the controls can be adjusted and the details on the screen scrutinized by the operator while the transducer is being held in position. Scanning animals secured in rows, as in a dairy barn, can be done by fastening the scanner to a portable cart (pg 133).

Preparing a large animal for transrectal ultrasound examination (restraint, evacuation of rectum) is similar to preparing for transrectal palpation (pg 130). Fecal material can cause distortions on the ultrasound image and must be removed. A pronounced shadow extending from the upper edge of the image may be due to intervening fecal matter. Each operator should develop a systematic procedure, depending on whether selected areas or the entire tract is of interest at any given examination. During the examination, the viewing screen is the center of visual attention. At the same time, the location and orientation of the transducer and the resulting field of view are considered.

The water bath technique is important for training or research (pg 136). The standoff technique can be used when the transducer face is too close to the needed tissue information (pg 137). Commercially available standoff material can be mounted or held between the transducer face and the contact area. Simulated structures, contrast media, and markers can be used as adjuncts to ultrasonically based research (pg 140). Ultrasonically guided instrumentation is becoming popular in animal reproduction, especially for transvaginal aspiration of follicular oocytes for in vitro fertilization work (pg 142).

9. Research Aspects (pgs 147 to 169)

In the short time that transrectal ultrasonic imaging of the reproductive tract has been used as a research tool, many discoveries have resulted, some of which would otherwise have escaped detection for many years (pg 147). Prior to the introduction of real-time ultrasonic imaging in animal reproduction research, the dynamic aspects of morphology were largely inaccessible. A dynamic event (e.g., ovulation) can be monitored in entirety by continuous observation (e.g., 30 min), or examinations can be done repeatedly over many days. Maximal research utilization of ultrasonography requires good equipment and examining conditions, keen observational skills, and creative utilization. The techniques of using simulating structures, marking specific areas, and guiding insertion devices (e.g., insemination pipette, biopsy or aspiration needle) illustrate how the power of ultrasonography can be even further extended. Furthermore, the technology adds a measure of excitement to research because of the ability to observe dynamic reproductive events as they occur, including events that were previously unknown.

Ovulation is a superb ultrasonic reference and end point (pg 148). Ovulation has the following advantages over the traditional reference point, estrus: 1) readily and objectively detected; 2) encompasses a narrow time-span; 3) represents a profound and central endocrinologic event; and 4) detection requires little additional time if the study involves ultrasonic examinations for other reasons. Other ovarian reference and end points that have become available solely through ultrasonography include the following: 1) day of emergence of a follicular wave, 2) day of divergence of follicles into dominant and subordinate categories, 3) beginning of regression of an anovulatory dominant follicle, and 4) beginning of morphologic luteolysis. Each of these characteristics will require a firm definition as part of the experimental protocol.

A discrete reference and end point that was unimaginable before the introduction of transrectal ultrasonography is the establishment of the time of embryonic death (pg 149). The embryonal heartbeat is obvious by Day 24, and detecting its cessation provides the scientist with one of the criteria used for death in adults. In addition to the above discrete end points, many quantitative end points have become available through the imaging technology. Included are the following: 1) diameter, area, or growth and regression rates of follicles;

2) diameter or growth rate of the embryonic vesicle, embryo proper, and other measurable structures involving the conceptus; 3) diameter, area, or growth and regression rates of the corpus luteum; 4) heart rate; 5) rate of mobility of the embryonic vesicle in mares; 6) diameter or other measures of the uterus; and 7) height or other measures of fluid pockets in the uterus, vagina, and conceptus.

Scoring of end points is a useful technique for ultrasonic characteristics that are not conveniently amenable to conventional measuring techniques (pg 150). Scoring can be used, for example, for the relative amount of a substance that cannot be easily measured, such as intrauterine fluid and endometrial edema, or the extent of uterine contractions or changes in uterine shape. The scoring approach facilitates profiling or statistically analyzing changes during a defined time period, such as the estrous cycle. End points involving changes in number or frequency over time are also useful (pg 152). Centralization of events onto a normalized day scale (e.g., days of the interovulatory interval) are also efficient maneuvers for characterization and temporalization studies (pg 154).

In recent years, the following analytical techniques have been developed for processing ovarian follicular data: 1) grouping follicles according to size categories; 2) monitoring individual follicles from day to day (follicle-identity method; pg 158); 3) profiling follicles on the basis of diameter without regard to day-to-day identity (nonidentity method); 4) constructing mean profiles by means of centralization and normalization (pg 161); 5) mathematically detecting follicular waves by significant increases and decreases in follicle diameters in individual animals (pg 162); and 6) partitioning follicles into tiers of progressively decreasing diameters (tier method; pg 163).

Ultrasonic image information can be digitized and analyzed by computer (pg 164). Digitization is a procedure in which each pixel of an image is assigned a numeric value for brightness and location. Conversion of image information to numerical data allows the use of quantitative statistics for temporal characterizations or testing of hypotheses. However, the sophisticated processing does not eliminate bias. The operator retains the responsibility of selecting and delineating the areas to be processed, and these decisions are notoriously subject to bias. Computer analyses, therefore, can be dangerous and lull the operator into a false sense of well-being. Since it may not be practical to expose the computer to barn conditions, the image information may be stored with a high-resolution videotape system. The analogue format used on the videotape is then reconverted to the digitized format at the laboratory. Pixel analyses have been used to characterize the day-to-day changes in the intensity of echogenicity of the corpus luteum and to quantify changes in shape of the preovulatory follicle as ovulation approaches. The NIH image analysis system for MacIntosh computers is available without charge by electronic mail (e-mail) from the National Institutes of Health (pg 168). The program can acquire, display, edit, enhance, analyze, and print images.

Part Five

APPENDIX

SOURCE INFORMATION

The addresses and phone numbers listed below are those currently in the author's files. The market is volatile with turn-overs or discontinuations in availability and sources. Listing of an item or source does not represent an endorsement. If the representative for a country or area is not listed, the needed information can be obtained from the headquarters, if given.

Ultrasound Scanners and Supplies for Animals

Aloka

Aloka Co., LTD. (Headquarters)
6-22-1, Mure, Mitaka-shi
Tokyo, 181 Japan
Phone: 0422-45-5111

Corometrics Medical Systems, Inc. (USA representative)
61 Barnes Park Road North
Wallingford, Connecticut 06492-0333 USA
Phone: 203-265-5631; 800-243-3952
Fax: 203-949-1622

Instruments for Science and Medicine (E. Canada representative)
250 Rue Authier
St. Laurent, Quebec H4M 2C6 Canada
Phone: 514-744-2893
Fax: 514-744-2596

Omnium Medical Devices of Canada, Inc. (Ontario representative)
Unit 8, 75 East Beaver Creek Road
Richmond Hill, Ontario L4B 1K6 Canada
Phone: 905-886-2105
Fax: 905-886-2109

Overseas Monitor Corporation (W. Canada representative)
150-13151 Vanier Place
Richmond, British Columbia V6V 2J2 Canada
Phone: 604-270-7261; 800-663-6064
Fax: 604-270-4127

Ausonics

Universal Medical Systems
299 Adams Street
Bedford Hills, New York 10507 USA
Phones: 914-666-6200; 800-842-0607
Fax: 914-666-2454

Dynamic Imaging

Dynamic Imaging Ltd. (Headquarters)
Brucefield Industrial Park
Livingston, EH54 9DR Scotland UK
Phone: 0506-415282
Fax: 0506-410603

Dynamic Imaging (Germany representative)
Heiliger Weg 99
44141 Dortmund, Germany
Phone: 0231-52-89-41-42
Fax: 0231-52-89-43

Products Group International, Inc. (USA representative)
2805 Wilderness Place, Suite 900
Boulder, Colorado 80301 USA
Phone: 303-939-9380; 800-336-5299
Fax: 303-442-8159

Pie Medical

Pie Medical Equipment B.V. (Headquarters)
Philipsweg 1
6227AJ Maastricht Holland
Phone: 31-43-824600
Fax: 31-43-824601

Classic Medical Supply, Inc. (USA representative)
19900 Mona Road, Suite 105
Tequesta, Florida 33469 USA
Phones: 407-746-9527; 800-722-6838
Fax: 407-746-4212

SonoAce

Medison America, Inc.
5319 Randall Place
Freemont, California 94538 USA
Phone: 501-249-0140

Tokyo Keiki

Tokyo Keiki Co., LTD. (Headquarters)
16 Minami-Kamata
2-chome, Oh ta-ku
Tokyo, 144 Japan
Phone: 03-732-2111

Products Group International, Inc. (USA representative)
2805 Wilderness Place, Suite 900
Boulder, Colorado 80301 USA
Phone: 303-939-9380; 800-336-5299
Fax: 303-449-7605

Tokyo Keiki has discontinued their line of ultrasound scanners for animals.

Shimadzu

Universal Medical Supplies
299 Adams Street
Bedford Hills, New York 10507 USA
Phones: 914-666-6200; 800-842-0607
Fax: 914-666-2454

Ultra-Scan

Alliance Medical Inc. (Headquarters)
5919 Henri-Bourassa W., Suite 108
Montreal, Quebec H4R 1B7 Canada
Phone: 514-745-3777
Fax: 514-337-9242

TAC sales (USA representative)
1553 S. Highway 169, Suite A
Smithville, Missouri 64089 USA
Phones: 816-532-9977; 800-878-7226
Fax: 816-873-3223

Pameda Ag Basel (European representative)
Grabenackerstrasse 11
CH-4142 Müchenstein, Switzerland
Phone: 61-46-0997
Fax: 61-46-0993

Genesis (Doppler instruments)

Products Group International, Inc. (USA representative)
2805 Wilderness Place, Suite 900
Boulder, Colorado 80301 USA
Phone: 303-939-9380; 800-336-5299
Fax: 303-449-7605

Ultrasound-Guided Aspiration Equipment

Cook Australia (Headquarters)
12 Electronics Street
Bisbane Technological Park
Eight Mile Plains, Queensland 4113 Australia
Phone: 07-841-1188
Fax: 07-841-1288

Cook Veterinary Products (USA representative)
127 South Main Street
P.O. Box 266
Spencer, Indiana 47460 USA
Phone: 800-826-2380
Fax: 812-829-6535

Some ultrasound equipment suppliers also carry transvaginal aspiration equipment.

Ultrasound Phantoms

Gammex RMI
2500 West Beltline Highway
P.O. Box 620327
Middleton, Wisconsin 53562 USA
Phone: 608-831-1188; 800-426-6391
Fax: 608-836-9201

Some ultrasound equipment suppliers also carry phantoms.

Instructional Videotapes and Short Courses

American Institute of Ultrasound in Medicine
14750 Sweitzer Lane, Suite 100
Laurel, Maryland 20707-5906 USA
Phone: 301-498-4100; 800-638-5352
Fax: 301-498-4450

Equiservices Publishing
4343 Garfoot Road
Cross Plains, Wisconsin 53528 USA
Phone: 608-798-4910
Fax: 608-798-4910

Radiological Society of North America
Educational Materials
PO Box 5316
Oak Brook, Illinois 60522-5316 USA
Phone: 800-272-2920
Fax: 708-575-2910

Many veterinary schools and a few animal science departments offer short courses in multidisciplinary ultrasonography and a few have courses in equine reproductive ultrasonography (Colorado State University, 303-491-8373; Texas A & M University, 409-845-7731).

Carts

Wheelit, Inc.
P.O. Box 352800
Toledo, Ohio 43635-2800 USA
Phone: 800-523-7508
Fax: 419-531-6415

Some ultrasound equipment suppliers also have scanner carts.

Coupling Gel

Aqualon
1313 North Market Street, P.O. Box 8740
Wilmington, Delaware 19899 USA
Phone: 800-334-8426, Extension 6

Inquire about carboxy-methyl-cellulose powder, Type 7H3-SF; 50 lb. bags.

Most ultrasound equipment suppliers also carry a gel, but in a more expensive prepared form.

NIH *Image*

Image can be obtained free of charge by e-mail, if access to Internet is available. The e-mail address is wayne@helix.nih.gov. The reply will be in three messages containing the program, manual, and source code. The messages will be in BinHex format and can be decoded using "Stuffit" 1.5.1. or a more recent version.

Image can also be purchased for approximately $100 on a diskette using order number PB93-504868 from the following address:

National Information Service
5285 Port Royal Road
Springfield, Virginia 22161 USA
Phone: 703-487-4650

Since *Image* is in the public domain, it may be freely copied from other users or from Macintosh bulletin boards and user-group libraries.

BIBLIOGRAPHY

NOTE: Pages where reference is cited are given at the end of each reference.

1. **Adams** GP, Griffin PG, Ginther OJ. 1989. In situ morphologic dynamics of ovaries, uterus, and cervix in llamas. *Biol. Reprod.* 41:551-558. (cited on pgs 15, 21)

2. **Adams** GP, Kastelic JP, Bergfelt DR, Ginther OJ. 1987. Effect of uterine inflammation and ultrasonically-detected uterine pathology on fertility in the mare. *J. Reprod. Fert., Suppl.* 35:445-454. (cited on pg 13)

3. **Adams** GP, Matteri RL, Kastelic JP, Ko JCH, Ginther OJ. 1992. Associations between surges of follicle-stimulating hormone and the emergence of follicular waves in heifers. *J. Reprod. Fert.* 94:177-188. (cited on pgs 16, 22)

4. **Adams** GP, Plotka ED, Asa CS, Ginther OJ. 1991. Feasibility of characterizing reproductive events in large nondomestic species by transrectal ultrasonic imaging. *Zoo Anim. Biol.* 10:247-259. (cited on pg 16)

5. **Adams** GP, Sumar J, Ginther OJ. 1990. Effects of lactational and reproductive status on ovarian follicular waves in llamas (Lama glama). *J. Reprod. Fert.* 90:535-545. (cited on pgs 15, 21)

6. **Adams** GP, Sumar J, Ginther OJ. 1991. Form and function of the corpus luteum in llamas. *Anim. Reprod. Sci.* 24:127-138. (cited on pg 16)

7. **Alasaarela** E, Koivukangas J. 1990. Evaluation of image quality of ultrasound scanners in medical diagnostics. *J. Ultrasound Med.* 9:23-34. (cited on pgs 99, 103)

8. **Allen** JK, Kramer RW. 1993. Enhanced sonographic visualization of biopsy needles. *Vet. Radiol. and Ultrasound* 34:359-360. (cited on pg 144)

9. **Athey** PA, McClendon L. 1983. *Diagnostic Ultrasound for Radiographers*. Multi-Media Publishing, Inc., Denver, Colorado. (cited on pg 18)

10. **Bamber** JC, Hill CR, King JA, Dunn F. 1979. Ultrasonic propagation through fixed and unfixed tissues. *Ultrasound in Med. and Biol.* 5:159-165. (cited on pg 103)

11. **Barr** F. 1990. *Diagnostic Ultrasound in the Dog and the Cat*. Blackwell Scientific Publications, London. (cited on pg 24)

12. **Baum** D. 1993. Visual analysis software opens window on medicine. *Infoworld*, Oct. 18, p 66. (cited on pgs 125, 169)

13. **Beal** WE, Edwards RB, Kearnan JM. 1989. Use of B-mode, linear array ultrasonography for evaluating the technique of bovine artificial insemination. *J. Diary Sci.* 72:2198-2202. (cited on pg 15)

14. **Bergfelt** DR, Ginther OJ. 1992. Relationships between circulating concentrations of FSH and follicular waves during early pregnancy in mares. *J. Equine Vet. Sci.* 12:274-279. (cited on pgs 16, 22, 157)

15. **Bergfelt** DR, Pierson RA, Ginther OJ. 1989. Resurgence of the primary corpus luteum during pregnancy in the mare. *Anim. Reprod. Sci.* 21:261-270. (cited on pg 21)

16. **Biller** DS, Myer W. 1988. Ultrasound scanning of superficial structures using an ultrasound standoff pad. *Vet. Radiol.* 29:138-142. (cited on pg 137)

17. **Bingham** CM, Wilson PR, Davies AS. 1990. Real-time ultrasonography for pregnancy diagnosis and estimation of fetal age in farmed red deer. *Vet. Rec.* 126:102-106. (cited on pg 15)

18. **Blackwell** R. 1988. Safety of diagnostic ultrasound. In: *Practical Ultrasound.* Edited by Lerski RA. IRL Press, Washington DC. pp 231-240. (cited on pg 26)

19. **Bonafos** LD, Kot K, Ginther OJ. 1995. Physical characteristics of the uterus during the bovine estrous cycle and early pregnancy. *Theriogenology* (submitted). (cited on pgs 17, 151)

20. **Bondestam** S, Alitali I, Karkkainen M. 1983. Real-time ultrasound pregnancy diagnosis in the bitch. *J. Sm. Anim. Pract.* 24:145-151. (cited on pgs 12, 139)

21. **Botero** O, Martinat-Botté F, Bariteau F. 1985. Use of ultrasound scanning in swine for detection of pregnancy and some pathological conditions. *Theriogenology* 26:267-278. (cited on pg 139)

22. **Boyd** JS, Omran SN. 1991. Diagnostic ultrasonography of the bovine female reproductive tract. *In Practice* 13:109-118. (cited on pg 24)

23. **Brück** I, Raun K, Synnestvedt B, Greve T. 1992. Follicle aspiration in the mare using a transvaginal ultrasound-guided technique. *Equine Vet. J.* 24:58-59. (cited on pgs 16, 143)

24. **Buckrell** BC, Bonnett BN, Johnson WH. 1986. The use of a real-time ultrasound rectally for early pregnancy diagnosis in sheep. *Theriogenology* 25:665-673. (cited on pg 14)

25. **Bushong** SC, Archer BR. 1991. *Diagnostic Ultrasound: Physics, Biology, and Instrumentation.* Mosby Year Book, St. Louis. pp 143-154. (cited on pgs 25, 26, 27, 29, 33, 39, 45, 48, 75, 81, 99)

26. **Carnevale** EM, Ginther OJ. 1993. Use of linear ultrasonic transducer for the transvaginal aspiration and transfer of oocytes in the mare. *J. Equine Vet. Sci.* 13:331-333. (cited on pgs 143, 144)

27. **Carnevale** EM, Ginther OJ. 1994. Defective oocytes as a cause of subfertility in old mares. *Int. Symp. on Equine Reprod.* (in press). (cited on pg 22)

28. **Cartee** RE. 1980. Diagnostic ultrasonography. *Mod. Vet. Prac.* 61:744-747. (cited on pgs 12, 17)

29. **Cartee** RE. 1980. Ultrasonography: A new diagnostic technique for veterinary medicine. *Vet. Med./Sm. Anim. Clin.* 75:1524-1533. (cited on pgs 12, 17)

30. **Cartee** RE, Powe TA, Jr., Ayer RL. 1985. Ultrasonographic detection of pregnancy in sows. *Mod. Vet. Pract.* 66:23-26. (cited on pg 13)

31. **Cartee** RE, Powe TA, Gray BW, Hudson RS, Kuhlers DL. 1986. Ultrasonographic evaluation of normal boar testicles. *Amer. J. Vet. Res.* 47:2543-2548. (cited on pg 14)

32. **Cartee** RE, Rowles T. 1983. Transabdominal sonographic evaluation of the canine prostate. *Vet. Radiol.* 24:156-164. (cited on pg 12)

33. **Chaffaux** S, Reddy GNS, Valon F, Thibier M. 1986. Transrectal real-time ultrasound scanning for diagnosing pregnancy and for monitoring embryonic mortality in dairy cattle. *Anim. Reprod. Sci.* 10:193-200. (cited on pg 13)

34. **Chaffaux** S, Valon F, Martinez J. 1982. Evolution de l'image échographique du produit de conception chez la vache. *Bull. Acad. Vét. de France* 55:213-221. (cited on pg 12)

35. **Chevalier** F, Palmer E. 1982. Ultrasonic echography in the mare. *J. Reprod. Fert., Suppl.* 32:423-430. (cited on pg 12)

36. **Cook** NL, Squires EL, Ray BS, Cook VM, Jasko DJ. 1992. Transvaginal ultrasonically guided follicular aspiration of equine oocytes: preliminary results. J. *Equine Vet. Sci.* 12:204-207. (cited on pgs 16, 143)

37. **Cross** DT, Ginther OJ. 1988. Uterine contractions in nonpregnant and early pregnant mares and jennies as determined by ultrasonography. *J. Anim. Sci.* 66:250-254. (cited on pgs 14, 21)

38. **Curran** S, Ginther OJ. 1989. Ultrasonic diagnosis of equine fetal sex by location of the genital tubercle. *J. Equine Vet. Sci.* 9:77-83. (cited on pg 15)

39. **Curran** S, Kastelic JP, Ginther OJ. 1989. Determining sex of the bovine fetus by ultrasonic assessment of the relative location of the genital tubercle. *Anim. Reprod. Sci.* 19:217-227. (cited on pg 15)

40. **Curran** S, Pierson RA, Ginther OJ. 1986. Embryonic loss and ultrasonic anatomy of the bovine conceptus on days 10 to 20. *J. Amer. Vet. Med. Assn.* 189:1289-1294. (cited on pg 13)

41. **Curran** S, Pierson RA, Ginther OJ. 1986. Ultrasonic anatomy of the bovine conceptus on days 20 to 60. *J. Amer. Vet. Med. Assn.*189:1295-1302. (cited on pg 13)

42. **Daels** PF, Ammon DC, Stabenfeldt GH, Liu IKM, Hughes JP, Lasley BL. 1991. Urinary and plasma estrogen conjugates, estradiol and estrone concentrations in nonpregnant and early pregnant mares. *Theriogenology* 35:1001-1017. (cited on pg 151)

43. **Davidson** AP, Nyland TG, Tsutsui T. 1986. Pregnancy diagnosis with ultrasound in the domestic cat. *Vet. Radiol.* 27:109-114. (cited on pgs 14, 139)

44. **Deichert** U, Schief R, van de Sandt M, Juhnke I. 1989. Transvaginal hysterosalpingo-contrast-sonography (Hy-Co-Sy) compared with conventional tubal diagnostics. *Human Reprod.* 4:418-424. (cited on pg 141)

45. **DuBose** TJ. 1991. Computer software for obstetric sonography. In: *Diagnostic Medical Sonography*, Vol. I. Edited by Berman MC. J. B. Lippincott Co., Philadelphia. pp 573-581. (cited on pg 125)

46. **Evans** ACO, Adams GP, Rawlings NC. 1993. Prepubertal ovarian and endocrine changes preceding first ovulation in heifers. *J. Reprod. Fert.* 100:187-194. (cited on pg 16)

47. **Evans** JA. 1988. Pulse-echo ultrasound. In: *Practical Ultrasound.* Edited by Lerski RA. IRL Press, Washington, DC. pp 15-29. (cited on pg 27)

48. **Fish** P. 1990. *Physics and Instrumentation of Diagnostic Medical Ultrasound.* John Wiley & Sons, New York. (cited on pgs 26, 27, 81)

49. **Fissore** RA, Edmondson AJ, Pashen RL, BonDurant RH. 1986. The use of ultrasonography for the study of the bovine reproductive tract. II. Nonpregnant, pregnant, and pathological conditions of the uterus. *Anim. Reprod. Sci.* 12:167-177. (cited on pg 13)

50. **Fleischer** AC, Kepple DM. 1992. Transvaginal color duplex sonography: clinical potentials and limitations. *Seminars in Ultrasound, CT, and MRI* 13:69-80. (cited on pg 109)

51. **Ginther** OJ. 1983. Fixation and orientation of the early equine conceptus. *Theriogenology* 19:613-623. (cited on pgs 12, 20, 116)

52. **Ginther** OJ. 1983. Mobility of the early equine conceptus. *Theriogenology* 19:603-611. (cited on pgs 12, 20)

53. **Ginther** OJ. 1984. Mobility of twin embryonic vesicles in mares. *Theriogenology* 22:83-95. (cited on pg 20)

54. **Ginther** OJ. 1984. Postfixation embryo reduction in unilateral and bilateral twins in mares. *Theriogenology* 22:213-223. (cited on pg 20)

55. **Ginther** OJ. 1984. Ultrasonic evaluation of the reproductive tract of the mare: The singleton embryo. *J. Equine Vet. Sci.* 4:75-81. (cited on pgs 12, 13)

56. **Ginther** OJ. 1985. Dynamic physical interactions between equine embryo and uterus. *Equine Vet. J., Suppl.* 3:41-47. (cited on pgs 13, 140)

57. **Ginther** OJ. 1985. Embryonic loss in mares: Nature of loss after experimental induction by ovariectomy or prostaglandin F2α. *Theriogenology* 24:87-98. (cited on pgs 13, 20)

58. **Ginther** OJ. 1986. *Ultrasonic Imaging and Reproductive Events in the Mare*. Equiservices Publishing, 4343 Garfoot Road, Cross Plains, Wisconsin, USA. (cited on pgs 13, 25, 26, 27, 113, 143)

59. **Ginther** OJ. 1988. Ultrasonic imaging of ovarian follicles and corpora lutea. *Vet. Clin. No. Amer.: Equine Pract.* 4:197-213. (cited on pg 24)

60. **Ginther** OJ. 1989. The nature of embryo reduction in mares with twin conceptuses: Deprivation hypothesis. *Am. J. Vet. Res.* 50:45-53. (cited on pg 21)

61. **Ginther** OJ. 1993. A method for characterizing ultrasonically derived follicular data in heifers. *Theriogenology* 39:363-371. (cited on pg 158)

62. **Ginther** OJ. 1993. Equine fetal kinetics: Allantoic-fluid shifts and uterine-horn closures. *Theriogenology* 40:241-256. (cited on pgs 16, 22)

63. **Ginther** OJ. 1993. Major and minor waves during the equine estrous cycle. *J. Equine Vet. Sci.* 13:18-25. (cited on pgs 22, 157, 162)

64. **Ginther** OJ. 1994. Equine physical utero-fetal interactions: A challenge and a wonder for the practitioner. *J. Equine Vet. Sci.* 14:313-318. (cited on pgs 17, 82)

65. **Ginther** OJ. 1994. Research applications of ultrasonic imaging in reproductive biology: Update 1994. In: *Livestock Production in the 21st Century*. Edited by Thacker PA. University of Saskatchewan, Saskatoon, Saskatchewan, Canada. pp 133-145. (cited on pg 24)

66. **Ginther** OJ, Bergfelt DR, Leith GS, Scraba ST. 1985. Embryonic loss in mares: Incidence and ultrasonic morphology. *Theriogenology* 24:73-86. (cited on pgs 13, 20)

67. **Ginther** OJ, Bergfelt DR. 1992. Associations between FSH concentrations and major and minor follicular waves in pregnant mares. *Theriogenology* 38:807-821. (cited on pgs 16, 22, 157)

68. **Ginther** OJ, Bergfelt DR. 1992. Ultrasonic characterization of follicular waves in mares without maintaining identity of individual follicles. *J. Equine Vet. Sci.* 12:349-354. (cited on pg 162)

69. **Ginther** OJ, Bergfelt DR. 1993. Growth of follicles and concentrations of FSH during the equine estrous cycle. *J. Reprod. Fert.* 99:105-111. (cited on pg 163)

70. **Ginther** OJ, Carnevale EM, Bergfelt DR. 1993. Delay in emergence of the ovulatory follicular waves in old mares. *J. Equine Vet. Sci.* 13:75-79. (cited on pg 22)

71. **Ginther** OJ, Garcia MC, Bergfelt DR, Leith GS, Scraba ST. 1985. Embryonic loss in mares: Pregnancy rate, length of interovulatory intervals, and progesterone concentrations associated with loss during days 11 to 15. *Theriogenology* 24:409-417. (cited on pg 13)

72. **Ginther** OJ, Ginther MR. 1994. *Ultrasonic Imaging and Reproductive Events: The Power and Principles.* Videotape. Equiservices Publishing, 4343 Garfoot Road, Cross Plains, Wisconsin, USA. (cited on pg 24)

73. **Ginther** OJ, Griffin PG. 1993. Equine fetal kinetics: Presentation and location. *Theriogenology* 40:1-11. (cited on pg 16)

74. **Ginther** OJ, Griffin PG. 1994. Natural outcome and ultrasonic identification of equine fetal twins. *Theriogenology* 41:1193-1199. (cited on pgs 17, 22)

75. **Ginther** OJ, Knopf L, Kastelic JP. 1989. Temporal associations among ovarian events during bovine oestrous cycles with two and three follicular waves. *J. Reprod. Fert.* 87:223-230. (cited on pgs 157, 161)

76. **Ginther** OJ, Kot K, Wiltbank MC. 1995. Associations between emergence of follicular waves and fluctuations in FSH concentrations during the estrous cycle in ewes. *Theriogenology* 43:689-703 (cited on pgs 17, 22, 154, 155)

77. **Ginther** OJ, Kot K. 1994. Follicular dynamics during the ovulatory season in goats. *Theriogenology* 42:987-1001. (cited on pgs 17, 22, 147)

78. **Ginther** OJ, Pierson RA. 1983. Ultrasonic evaluation of the reproductive tract of the mare: Principles, equipment, and techniques. *J. Equine Vet. Sci.* 3:195-201. (cited on pg 12)

79. **Ginther** OJ, Pierson RA. 1984. Ultrasonic anatomy and pathology of the equine uterus. *Theriogenology* 21:505-515. (cited on pg 13)

80. **Ginther** OJ, Pierson RA. 1984. Ultrasonic anatomy of equine ovaries. *Theriogenology* 21:471-483. (cited on pg 13)

81. **Ginther** OJ, Pierson RA. 1984. Ultrasonic evaluation of the reproductive tract of the mare: Ovaries. *J. Equine Vet. Sci.* 4:11-16. (cited on pg 12)

82. **Goldberg** BB, Liu J-B. 1992. Endoluminal ultrasound: vascular and nonvascular. *Ultrasound Quart.* 9:245-270. (cited on pg 138)

83. **Goldstein** A. 1991. Physics of ultrasound. In: *Diagnostic Ultrasound, Vol. I.* Edited by Rumack CM, Wilson SR, Charboneau JW. Mosby Year Book, St. Louis. pp 2-18. (cited on pg 27)

84. **Griffin** PG, Ginther OJ. 1991. Dynamics of uterine diameter and endometrial morphology during the estrous cycle and early pregnancy in mares. *Anim. Reprod. Sci.* 25:133-142. (cited on pgs 15, 16, 21, 140)

85. **Griffin** PG, Ginther OJ. 1992. Research applications of ultrasonography in reproductive biology. *J. Anim. Sci.* 70:953-972. (cited on pgs 16, 24)

86. **Griffin** PG, Ginther OJ. 1993. Effects of the embryo on uterine morphology and function in mares. *Anim. Reprod. Sci.* 31:331-329. (cited on pg 22)

87. **Hayes** KEN, Pierson RA, Scraba ST, Ginther OJ. 1985. Effects of estrous cycle and season on ultrasonic uterine anatomy in mares. *Theriogenology* 24:465-477. (cited on pgs 20, 151)

88. **Hilpert** PL. 1991. Contrast agents in diagnostic ultrasound. In: *Diagnostic Ultrasound, Vol. I.* Edited by Rumack CM, Wilson SR, Charboneau JW. Mosby Year Book, St. Louis. pp 30-42. (cited on pg 141)

89. **Hoppe** FE, Hager DA, Poulos PW, Ekman S, Lindgren PG. 1986. A comparison of manual and automatic ultrasound-guided biopsy techniques. *Vet. Radiol.* 27:99-101. (cited on pg 143)

90. **Inaba** T, Matsui N, Shimizu R, Imori T. 1984. Use of echography in bitches for detection of ovulation and pregnancy. *Vet. Rec.* 115:276-277. (cited on pg 13)

91. **Inaba** T, Nakazima Y, Matsui N, Imori T. 1983. Early pregnancy diagnosis in sows by ultrasonic linear electronic scanning. *Theriogenology* 20:97-101. (cited on pg 12)

92. **Irving** HC. 1988. Interventional ultrasound. In: *Practical Ultrasound.* Edited by Lerski RA. IRL Press, Washington DC. pp 217-229. (cited on pg 143)

93. **Kähn** W. 1989. Sonographic fetometry in the bovine. *Theriogenology* 31:1105-1121. (cited on pg 15)

94. **Kähn** W, Lcidl W, Rienmüller R. 1989. Die kammerung des rinderuterus während de Frühgravidität. *J. Vet. Med.* 36:641-652. (cited on pg 21)

95. **Kastelic** JP, Curran S, Pierson RA, Ginther OJ. 1988. Ultrasonic evaluation of the bovine conceptus. *Theriogenology* 29:39-54. (cited on pgs 14, 24)

96. **Kastelic** JP, Ginther OJ. 1989. Fate of conceptus and corpus luteum after induced embryonic loss in heifers. *J. Amer. Vet. Med. Assoc.* 194:922-928. (cited on pg 21)

97. **Khamis** HJ, Warner RW. 1991. Statistical methods in obstetric ultrasound. In: *Diagnostic Medical Sonography.* Vol. I. Edited by Berman MC. J. B. Lippincott Co., Philadelphia. pp 583-594. (cited on pg 147)

98. **Kito** S, Okuda K, Miyazawa K, Sato K. 1986. Study on the appearance of the cavity in the corpus luteum of cows by using ultrasonic scanning. *Theriogenology* 25:325-333. (cited on pg 13)

99. **Kremkau** FW. 1991. Biologic effects and safety. In: *Diagnostic Ultrasound.* Edited by Rumack CM, Wilson SR, Charboneau JW. Mosby Year Book, St. Louis. (cited on pg 26)

100. **Lavoir** MC, Taverne MAM. 1989. The diagnosis of pregnancy and pseudopregnancy, and the determination of foetal numbers of goats, by means of real-time ultrasound scanning. In: *Diagnostic Ultrasound and Animal Reproduction.* Edited by Taverne MAM, Willemse AH. Kluwer Academic Publishers, Boston. pp 89-96. (cited on pgs 24, 139)

101. **Leith** GS, Ginther OJ. 1984. Characterization of intrauterine mobility of the early conceptus. *Theriogenology* 22:401-408. (cited on pg 152)

102. **Little** TV, Woods GL. 1987. Ultrasonography of accessory sex glands in the stallion. *J. Reprod. Fert., Suppl.* 35:87-94. (cited on pg 14)

103. **Love** CC, Garcia MC, Riera FR, Kenney RM. 1990. Evaluation of measures taken by ultrasonography and calipers to estimate testicular volume and predict daily sperm output in the stallion. *J. Reprod. Fert., Suppl.* 44:99-105. (cited on pg 15)

104. **Mack** LA, Lee RA, Nyberg DA. 1991. Intraoperative sonography of the abdomen. In: *Diagnostic Ultrasound.* Edited by Rumack CM, Wilson SR, Charboneau JW. Mosby Year Book, St. Louis. pp 492-504. (cited on pg 138)

105. **Malmgren** L, Sussemilch B-I. 1992. Ultrasonography as a diagnostic tool in a stallion with seminal vesiculitis: A case report. *Theriogenology* 37:935-938. (cited on pg 16)

106. **McDicken** WN. 1991. *Diagnostic Ultrasonics: Principles and Use of Instruments.* 3rd Ed. Churchill Livingstone, New York City. (cited on pgs 27, 35, 53, 81, 87, 113, 127, 131, 137)

107. **McDicken** WN. 1991. Quality assurance for echo imaging. In: *Diagnostic Ultrasonics: Principles and Use of Instruments,* 3rd Ed. Churchill Livingstone, New York. pp 323-328. (cited on pg 99)

108. **McGladdery** AL. 1993. Doppler ultrasound studies of umbilical circulation. *J. Equine Vet. Sci.* 13:622. (cited on pg 109)

109. **McKinnon** AO, Squires EL, Voss JL. 1987. Ultrasonic evaluation of the mare's reproductive tract-Part I. *Compend. Cont. Ed. Pract. Vet.* 9:335-345. (cited on pg 24)

110. **McKinnon** AO, Squires EL, Voss JL. 1987. Ultrasonic evaluation of the mare's reproductive tract-Part II. *Compend. Cont. Ed. Pract. Vet.* 9:472-480. (cited on pg 24)

111. **McKinnon** AO, Voss JL, Squires EL, Carnevale EM. 1993. Diagnostic ultrasonography. In: *Equine Reproduction.* Edited by McKinnon AO, Voss JL. Lea & Febiger, Philadelphia. pp 266-302. (cited on pg 24)

112. **Müller** E, Wittkowski G. 1986. Visualization of male and female characteristics of bovine fetuses by real-time ultrasonics. *Theriogenology* 22:571-580. (cited on pg 14)

113. **Norman** ST, Fields MJ. 1993. Ultrasound-guided cannulation of the caudal vena cava in the bovine for selective sampling of ovarian effluent. *Theriogenology* 39:691-701. (cited on pg 16)

114. **O'Grady** JP, Yeager CH, Findleton L, Brown J, Esra G. 1981. In utero visualization of the fetal horse by ultrasonic scanning. *Equine Pract.* 3:45-49. (cited on pgs 12, 139)

115. **O'Neal** GE. 1993. Ultrasonography in Camelids: A management tool. *The Ultrasound Review,* Tequesta, Florida, USA. (cited on pg 139)

116. **Okano** A, Tomizuka T. 1987. Ultrasonic observation of postpartum uterine involution in the cow. *Theriogenology* 27:369-376 (cited on pg 14).

117. **Palmer** E, Driancourt MA. 1980. Use of ultrasonic echography in equine gynecology. *Theriogenology* 13:203-216. (cited on pgs 12, 17)

118. **Pawshe** CH, Appa Rao KBC, Totey SM. 1994. Ultrasonographic imaging to monitor early pregnancy and embryonic development in the buffalo (Bubalus bubalis). *Theriogenology* 41:697-709. (cited on pg 17)

119. **Pechman** RD, Eilts BE. 1987. B-mode ultrasonography of the bull testicle. *Theriogenology* 27:431-441. (cited on pg 14)

120. **Penninck** DG, Crystal MA, Matz ME, Pearson SH. 1993. The technique of percutaneous ultrasound guided fine-needle aspiration biopsy and automated microcore biopsy in small animal gastrointestinal diseases. *Vet. Radiol. and Ultrasound* 34:433-436. (cited on pg 143)

121. **Pierson** RA, Adams GP. 1994. Computer-assisted analysis of ultrasonographic images of dominant anovulatory and ovulatory follicles in heifers. *Theriogenology* 41:275 (abstract). (cited on pg 167)

122. **Pierson** RA, Ginther OJ. 1984. Ultrasonography for detection of pregnancy and study of embryonic development in heifers. *Theriogenology* 22:225-233. (cited on pg 13)

123. **Pierson** RA, Ginther OJ. 1984. Ultrasonography of the bovine ovary. *Theriogenology* 21:495-504. (cited on pg 13)

124. **Pierson** RA, Ginther OJ. 1985. Ultrasonic evaluation of the corpus luteum of the mare. *Theriogenology* 23:795-806. (cited on pgs 13, 20, 153)

125. **Pierson** RA, Ginther OJ. 1985. Ultrasonic evaluation of the preovulatory follicle in the mare. *Theriogenology* 24:359-368. (cited on pg 13)

126. **Pierson** RA, Ginther OJ. 1986. Ovarian follicular populations during early pregnancy in heifers. *Theriogenology* 26:649-658. (cited on pg 20)

127. **Pierson** RA, Ginther OJ. 1987. Follicular population dynamics during the estrous cycle of the mare. *Anim. Reprod. Sci.* 14:219-231. (cited on pg 20)

128. **Pierson** RA, Ginther OJ. 1987. Ultrasonographic appearance of the bovine uterus during the estrous cycle. *J. Amer. Vet. Med. Assoc.* 190:995-1001. (cited on pgs 14, 20, 151, 152)

129. **Pierson** RA, Ginther OJ. 1988. Ultrasonic imaging of the ovaries and uterus in cattle. *Theriogenology* 29:21-37. (cited on pgs 14, 21, 24)

130. **Pierson** RA, Kastelic JP, Ginther OJ. 1988. Basic principles and techniques for transrectal ultrasonography in cattle and horses. *Theriogenology* 29:3-20. (cited on pgs 24, 138)

131. **Pieterse** MC, Kappen KA, Kruip ThAM, Taverne MAM. 1988. Aspiration of bovine oocytes during transvaginal ultrasound scanning of the ovaries. *Theriogenology* 30:751-762. (cited on pgs 14, 143)

132. **Pipers** FS, Adams-Brendemuehl CS. 1984. Techniques and applications of transabdominal ultrasonography in the pregnant mare. *J. Amer. Vet. Med. Assoc.* 185:766-771. (cited on pg 139)

133. **Poffenbarger** EM, Feeney DA. 1986. Use of gray-scale ultrasonography in the diagnosis of reproductive disease in the bitch: 18 cases (1981-84). *J. Amer. Vet. Med. Assoc.* 189:90-95. (cited on pg 14)

134. **Powis** RL. 1986. Ultrasound science for the veterinarian. *Vet. Clin. No. Amer.:Equine Pract.* 2:3-27. (cited on pg 33)

135. **Powis** RL. 1990. Transducing frequencies galore. *The Ultrasound Review*, Tequesta, Florida, USA. (cited on pg 40)

136. **Powis** RL. 1990. Harvesting preferred transducer frequencies. *The Ultrasound Review*, Tequesta, Florida, USA. (cited on pg 40)

137. **Radiation Measurements, Inc**. 1994. *The QA Cookbook for Ultrasound.* Gammex RMI, Middleton, Wisconsin, USA. (cited on pg 99)

138. **Rantanen** NW, Ewing RL. 1981. Principles of ultrasound application in animals. *Vet. Radiol.* 22:196-203. (cited on pg 23)

139. **Rantanen** NW, Torbeck RL, DuMond SS. 1982. Early pregnancy diagnosis in the mare using transrectal ultrasound scanning techniques: a preliminary report. *J. Equine Vet. Sci.* 2:27-29. (cited on pg 12)

140. **Reading** CC, Charboneau JW. 1991. Ultrasound-guided biopsy of the abdomen and pelvis. In: *Diagnostic Ultrasound.* Edited by Rumack CM, Wilson SR, Charboneau JW. Mosby Year Book, St. Louis. pp 429-442. (cited on pg 143)

141. **Reef** VB. 1991. The use of diagnostic ultrasound in the horse. *Ultrasound Quart.* 9:1-33. (cited on pg 24)

142. **Reeves** JJ, Rantanen NW, Hauser M. 1984. Transrectal real-time ultrasound scanning of the cow reproductive tract. *Theriogenology* 21:485-494. (cited on pg 13)

143. **Reisner** SA, Shapiro JR, Schwarz KQ, Meltzer RS. 1988. Sonication of echocontrast agents: a standardized and reproducible method. *J. Cardiovasc. Ultrasonography* 7:273-276. (cited on pg 141)

144. **Russel** AJF. 1989. The application of real-time ultrasonic scanning in commercial sheep, goats and cattle production enterprises. In: *Diagnostic Ultrasound and Animal Reproduction.* Edited by Taverne MAM, Willemse AH. Kluwer Academic Publishers, Boston. pp 73-87. (cited on pgs 24, 139)

145. **Ryan** DP, Yaakub H, Harrington D, Lynch PB. 1994. Follicular development during early pregnancy and the estrous cycle of the sow. *Theriogenology* 42:623-632. (cited on pg 17)

146. **Sarti** DA, Sample WF. 1980. *Diagnostic Ultrasound; Text and Cases.* G. K. Hall and Co., Boston. (cited on pg 78)

147. **Savio** JD, Kennan L, Boland MP, Roche JF. 1988. Pattern of growth of dominant follicles during the oestrus cycle in heifers. *J. Reprod. Fert.* 83:663-671. (cited on pgs 14, 21)

148. **Schrick** FN, Surface RA, Pritchard JY, Dailey RA, Townsend EC, Inskeep EK. 1993. Ovarian structures during the estrous cycle and early pregnancy in ewes. *Biol. Reprod.* 49:1133-1140. (cited on pg 16)

149. **Schwimer** SR, Rothman CM, Lebovic J, Oye DM. 1984. The effect of ultrasound coupling gels on sperm motility in vitro. *Fert. and Steril.* 42:946-947. (cited on pg 143)

150. **Simpson** DJ, Greenwood RES, Ricketts SW, Rossdale PD, Sanderson M, Allen WR. 1982. Use of ultrasound echography for early diagnosis of single and twin pregnancy in the mare. *J. Reprod. Fert., Suppl.* 3:431-439. (cited on pg 12)

151. **Sirois** J, Ball BA, Fortune JE. 1989. Patterns of growth and regression of ovarian follicles during the oestrous cycle and after hemiovariectomy in mares. *Equine Vet. J., Suppl.* 8:43-48. (cited on pg 15)

152. **Sirois** J, Fortune JE. 1988. Ovarian follicular dynamics during the estrous cycle in heifers monitored by real-time ultrasonography. *Biol. Reprod.* 39:308-317. (cited on pgs 14, 21)

153. **Soede** NM, Kemp B. 1993. In synchronized pigs, the duration of ovulation is not affected by insemination and is not a determinant for early embryonic diversity. *Theriogenology* 39:1043-1053. (cited on pg 16)

154. **Spaulding** KA. 1992. Use of an ultrasound phantom. *Vet. Radiol. and Ultrasound* 33:199-200. (cited on pg 103)

155. **Squires** EL, McKinnon AO, Shideler RK. 1988. Use of ultrasonography in reproductive management of mares. *Theriogenology* 29:55-70. (cited on pg 24)

156. **Szenci** O, Piros A, Kovács L. 1990. Early bovine pregnancy diagnosis by a battery operated portable ultrasonic scanner the "Ultra-scan". *16th World Buiatnic Congr.*, Salvador, Brasil. pp 219-223. (cited on pg 111)

157. **Taverne** MAM. 1989. The use of linear array real-time ultrasonography for pregnancy diagnosis in pigs. In: *Diagnostic Ultrasound and Animal Reproduction.* Edited by Taverne MAM, Willemse AH. Kluwer Academic Publishers, Boston. pp 97-103. (cited on pgs 24, 139)

158. **Taverne** MAM, van Oord HA. 1989. Accuracy of pregnancy diagnosis in dogs by means of linear-array ultrasound scanning. In: *Diagnostic Ultrasound and Animal Reproduction.* Edited by Taverne MAM, Willemse AH. Kluwer Academic Publishers, Boston. pp 105-110. (cited on pgs 24, 139)

159. **Taverne** MAM, Willemse AH, (editors). 1989. *Diagnostic Ultrasound and Animal Reproduction.* Kluwer Academic Publishers, Boston. (cited on pgs 15, 24)

160. **Taylor** KJW, Burns PN, Wells PNT, Conway DI, Hull MGR. 1985. Ultrasound Doppler flow studies of the ovarian and uterine arteries. *Br. J. Obstet. Gynec.* 92:240-246. (cited on pg 109)

161. **Thomenius** KE, Lewin PA. 1991. Ultrasound bioeffects 1991: an update. *Ultrasound Quart.* 9:111-137. (cited on pg 26)

162. **Thrall** DE. 1991. Editorial. *Vet. Radiol.* 32:266-267. (cited on pg 24)

163. **Tom** JW, Pierson RA, Adams GP. 1994. Ultrasonographic image attributes of bovine ovarian follicles. In: *Livestock Production in the 21st Century:* Edited by Thacker PA. University of Saskatchewan, Saskatoon, Saskatchewan, Canada. (Abstract 94P-36). (cited on pg 167)

164. **Townson** DH, Ginther OJ. 1987. Duration and pattern of follicular evacuation during ovulation in the mare. *Anim. Reprod. Sci.* 15:131-138. (cited on pgs 14, 21)

165. **Townson** DH, Ginther OJ. 1989. Size and shape changes in the preovulatory follicle in mares based on digital analysis of ultrasonic images. *Anim. Reprod. Sci.* 21:63-71. (cited on pgs 15, 164, 166)

166. **Townson** DH, Ginther OJ. 1989. Ultrasonic characterization of follicular evacuation during ovulation and fate of the discharged follicular fluid in mares. *Anim. Reprod. Sci.* 20:131-141. (cited on pg 21)

167. **Townson** DH, Ginther OJ. 1989. Ultrasonic echogenicity of developing corpora lutea in pony mares. *Anim. Reprod. Sci.* 20:143-153. (cited on pgs 15, 164)

168. **Waite** LR, Ford SP, Young DF, Conley AJ. 1990. Use of ultrasonic doppler waveforms to estimate changes in uterine artery blood flow and vessel compliance. *J. Anim. Sci.* 68:2450-2458. (cited on pg 109)

169. **Wani** GM. 1981. Ultrasonic pregnancy diagnosis in sheep and goats - a review. *World Rev. Anim. Prod.* 17:43-48. (cited on pg 139)

170. **Weber** JA, Hilt CJ, Woods GL. 1988. Ultrasonographic appearance of bull accessory sex glands. *Theriogenology* 29:1347-1355. (cited on pg 15)

171. **Weber** JA, Woods GL. 1991. A technique for transrectal ultrasonography of stallions during ejaculation. *Theriogenology* 36:831-837. (cited on pg 16)

172. **Wells** PNT. 1993. Ultrasonic opportunities. *J. Ultrasound Med.* 12:1-9. (cited on pg 40)

173. **White** IR, Russel AJF, Fowler DG. 1984. Real-time scanning in the diagnosis of pregnancy and the determination of foetal numbers in sheep. *Vet. Rec.* 115:140-143. (cited on pgs 13, 139)

174. **Wicks** JD, Howe KS. 1983. *Fundamentals of Ultrasonic Technique.* Year Book Medical Publishers, Inc. Chicago. (cited on pg 78)

175. **Williamson** P, Gales NJ, Lister S. 1990. Use of real-time B-mode ultrasound for pregnancy diagnosis and measurement of fetal growth rate in captive bottlenose dolphins (Tursiops truncatus). *J. Reprod. Fert.* 88:543-548. (cited on pg 15)

176. **Winsberg** F, Cooperberg PL. 1982. *Real-Time Ultrasonography*. Churchill Livingstone, New York City. (cited on pgs 18, 81)

177. **Wrigley** RH. 1992. Abdominal ultrasonography in small animal veterinary practice. *Ultrasound Quart.* 10:155-183. (cited on pgs 24, 139)

178. **Zagzebski** J. 1983. Images and artifacts. In: *Textbook of Diagnostic Ultrasound.* Edited by Hagen-Ansert S. C. V. Mosby Co., St. Louis. (cited on pg 78)

179. **Zagzebski** J. 1983. Pulse-echo ultrasound instrumentation. In: *Textbook of Diagnostic Ultrasound.* Edited by Hagen-Ansert S. C. V. Mosby, St. Louis. (cited on pgs 76, 87, 94, 95)

SUBJECT INDEX